Dental Management of the Pregnant Patient

Dental Management of the Pregnant Patient

Edited by

Christos A. Skouteris, DMD, PhD

Clinical Assistant Professor
Department of Oral and Maxillofacial Surgery
University of Michigan School of Dentistry
and
Department of Surgery
Section of Oral and Maxillofacial Surgery
University of Michigan School of Medicine
Ann Arbor, MI, USA

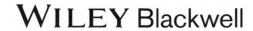

Registered Office
John Wiley & Sons, Inc., 111 River Street, Hoboken, NJ 07030, USA

Editorial Office
111 River Street, Hoboken, NJ 07030, USA

For details of our global editorial offices, customer services, and more information about Wiley products visit us at www.wiley.com.

Wiley also publishes its books in a variety of electronic formats and by print-on-demand. Some content that appears in standard print versions of this book may not be available in other formats.

Library of Congress Cataloging-in-Publication Data

Names: Skouteris, Christos A. (Christos Antonios), 1952– editor.
Title: Dental management of the pregnant patient / [edited] by Christos A. Skouteris.
Description: Hoboken, NJ : Wiley, 2018. | Includes bibliographical references and index. |
Identifiers: LCCN 2017052566 (print) | LCCN 2017053212 (ebook) | ISBN 9781119286578 (pdf) |
    ISBN 9781119286585 (epub) | ISBN 9781119286592 (oBook) | ISBN 9781119286561 (paperback)
Subjects: | MESH: Dental Care | Pregnancy | Pregnancy Complications
Classification: LCC RG551 (ebook) | LCC RG551 (print) | NLM WU 29 | DDC 618.2–dc23
LC record available at https://lccn.loc.gov/2017052566

Cover Design: Wiley
Cover Image: (Main) © skynesher/Gettyimages; (Top left) Courtesy of Christos A. Skouteris; (Top middle and right) Courtesy of Brent Ward

Set in 10/12pt Warnock by SPi Global, Pondicherry, India
Printed and bound in Singapore by Markono Print Media Pte Ltd

10 9 8 7 6 5 4 3 2 1

Dedications

In loving memory of my parents Antonios C. Skouteris, MD (1915–2008), Obstetrician-Gynecologist, and Maria A. Skouteris, CRN, (1918–1997), Chief Maternity Nurse.

To my family Kiki, Konstantinos, Eleni, Milou, Jolie, Perry, and Regina for their unconditional love and support.

To my mentor, George C. Sotereanos, DMD, MS, Oral and Maxillofacial Surgeon, a man of few words but with a wealth of experience and wisdom.

Contents

Preface

Pregnancy is a unique and momentous experience in a woman's life. As such, a comprehensive approach to the management of oral health problems that a woman may face during gestation becomes a necessity. My interest in embarking on the preparation of this book has three sources. First, the influence from my family environment. Both my parents were healthcare practitioners who worked in the area of obstetrics and gynecology throughout their professional lives. At an early age, I recall often listening with interest to long discussions on their experiences with pregnant patients. I started to realize the challenges that they had to face and I came to appreciate how deeply they cared about both the mother and the newborn child. In later years, as a dental student, I used to assist in the delivery room and in gynecologic surgical procedures and witnessed the miracle of childbirth. Although I had already made my career choice, I developed an interest in the care of the pregnant patient as a result of my early exposure to the intricacies of gestation. This interest was further augmented when I provided secretarial assistance to my father during his writing of two textbooks, one on menstruation and the other, a two-volume textbook on obstetrics and gynecology. Through my involvement in these projects, I learned a lot about the complexity of maternal physiology, the pathological conditions of pregnancy, and the potential risks that may complicate labor and delivery. It is only unfortunate that my father never had the opportunity to see his work published.

Then came the opportunity to provide surgical services to pregnant women during my academic and professional career as an oral and maxillofacial surgeon. Caring for pregnant women is an inimitable experience because in reality care is provided to two individuals, the mother and fetus. Even simple interventions may play an important role in achieving a successful outcome during dental treatment of an expectant woman and may prevent future implications on the quality of life of both mother and newborn. The well-being of both has to be the primary concern of the health provider.

Refreshing and updating my knowledge of the surgical management of the pregnant patient was dictated by the fact that proper care must be provided while assuring the safety of the mother and unborn child. Through my interaction with pregnant patients, I recognized that the management of their health issues needed to be urgent and decisive, often requiring a very thorough multidisciplinary intervention by a team of experienced professionals.

Finally, my pursuit of knowledge in the management of the pregnant patient showed that a more broad and systematic view on the treatment of maternal oral health issues was required. There are noble efforts in the literature to address the subject of oral health maintenance during pregnancy, but an in-depth approach is needed in view of recently published research data and advances in treatment modalities in many of the disciplines of medicine and dentistry that have a direct bearing upon the management of maternal morbidity. Moreover, there is insufficient discussion in the dental literature on the medical, obstetric, and gynecologic emergencies or familiarization of the oral health professional with the appropriate response in such circumstances. The importance of discussing with other specialists, in a holistic approach, the systemic and oral health problems during pregnancy is amply emphasized in this book, since the complexity of the pregnant state and maternal health management provide the perfect grounds for developing interprofessional collaboration. An interprofessional approach to the pregnant patient's needs leads to decisions that safeguard the safety and quality of life of the patient and fetus, while always considering and respecting patient autonomy. The decisions that are made can have a far-reaching impact on the immediate family and social environment of the pregnant patient.

The book also addresses the all-important issue of preparing for unexpected events. Many nonphysician public safety groups (paramedics, firefighters, police) have training in the handling of a prehospital event such as maternal cardiac arrest, impeding labor, and even on-scene delivery. There is practically no mention of such an event and its management in the dental literature related to care of the pregnant patient. Cardiac arrest during pregnancy and prehospital (on-scene) delivery in the dental office can be a potentially real situation and should be given its due attention. All these topics are discussed in the book and are supported by time-honored, recent, and current literature resources, quick-reference tables, and illustrations.

The book's intended readership includes dental and dental hygiene students, general dentists, dental hygienists, dental faculty, oral and maxillofacial surgeons, and specialized dentists in other disciplines of dentistry. This book could also be a useful reference source for physicians in the practice of general and family medicine.

I am indebted to the chapter contributors for embracing this project with warmth and enthusiasm and for offering their valuable input in the fields of their interest and expertise.

September 2017
Christos A. Skouteris,
DMD, PhD
Ann Arbor, Michigan

Acknowledgments

The editor wishes to acknowledge Mr Niles N. Mayrand, BBA, CMP, Manager, Clinical Simulation Center, Department of Learning Health Sciences, University of Michigan School of Medicine, for his assistance in the preparation of the simulated spontaneous vaginal delivery; Dr Andrew Beech, Oral and Maxillofacial Surgical Resident, for compiling the clinical information on the trauma cases; and Dr Kyriaki Marti for offering her artistic talent in the making of Figures 8.2 (a) and (b), 9.1, 9.2, and 9.3.

I would also like to thank my editor from Wiley, Mrs Jayadivya Saiprasad, with whom I had the pleasure to interact in preparation of this book, for keeping me on the right track with her astute comments and valuable suggestions.

List of Contributors

Benjamin Craig Cornwall, DDS, FICD
Assistant Professor, Hospital Dentistry
Director of General Practice Residency
University of Michigan
Ann Arbor, MI, USA

Sean P. Edwards, DDS, MD, FACS, FRCD[C]
Chalmers J. Lyons Endowed Clinical
Professor of Oral and Maxillofacial Surgery
Associate Professor and Residency Program
Director
Department of Surgery
Section of Oral and Maxillofacial Surgery
Chief, Pediatric Oral and Maxillofacial Surgery
University of Michigan School of Medicine
Ann Arbor, MI, USA

Igor Makovey, DDS, MD
Chief Resident
Department of Surgery
Section of Oral and Maxillofacial Surgery
University of Michigan School of Medicine
Ann Arbor, MI, USA

Kyriaki C. Marti, DMD, MD, MHPE, PhD, FEBOMS
Clinical Assistant Professor
Department of Oral and Maxillofacial Surgery
Department of Periodontics and Oral
Medicine

Department of Cariology, Restorative
Sciences and Endodontics
University of Michigan School of Dentistry
Ann Arbor, MI, USA

James Murphy BDS, MB, BCh, FFD
Attending Oral and Maxillofacial Surgeon
John H. Stroger Jr Hospital of Cook County
Chicago, IL, USA

Brent B. Ward, DDS, MD, FACS
Associate Professor and Chair
Department of Oral and Maxillofacial
Surgery
University of Michigan School of Dentistry
Section Head, Oral and Maxillofacial
Surgery/Hospital Dentistry
Department of Surgery, and Fellowship
Program Director
Oral/Head and Neck Oncology and
Microvascular Reconstructive Surgery
University of Michigan School of Medicine
Ann Arbor, MI, USA

1

Ethical Issues in the Treatment of the Pregnant Patient

Christos A. Skouteris

Ethical principles and the rights of the mother and fetus for the provision of proper medical and dental care are closely inter-twined. These principles are based on the fact that care is actually provided to two indi-viduals. Since the mother is the life support of the fetus, the medical and dental status of the mother should be optimized during preg-nancy. Therefore, necessary medical and dental treatment should not be denied to any female patient because of pregnancy.

Dental procedures, however minor, are associated with increased patient anxiety levels, the need for imaging, and the admin-istration of medications. For these reasons, elective dental procedures should be post-poned until postpartum. However, when a pregnant patient is in need of emergency, preventive, or restorative treatment, the aforementioned reasons may force the den-tist to refuse treatment because of concern for the mother and the unborn child and the fear of liability and litigation if something happens to the pregnancy and the fetus. Denial of treatment, however, raises serious ethical issues. Thomas Raimann (2016), in response to the question whether it is ethical for dentists to refuse seeing pregnant women until after they give birth, laid out the ethical principles of the ADA Code of Ethics that particularly apply in the dental management of the pregnant patient (Box 1.1).

The principle of patient **Autonomy** (self-governance) **and Involvement** states that

"The dentist should inform the patient of the proposed treatment in a manner that allows the patient to become involved in treatment decisions." Patient involvement in treatment decisions is highly desirable and ethical; however, pregnant women who have medical needs during pregnancy should not be expected to weigh the risks and benefits when they have to decide whether to proceed with a proposed treatment whose impact on the fetus is unknown. This is an impossible demand; no one can weigh unknown risks and benefits. On the other hand, a straight denial of treatment by the dentist without patient involvement becomes a unilateral decision and thus ethically questionable.

The principle of **Nonmaleficence** (do no harm) expresses the concept that profes-sionals have a duty to protect the patient from harm. Under this principle, the dentist's pri-mary obligations include keeping knowledge and skills current. Denying treatment to a pregnant patient violates this principle in the sense that it is evidence of lack of knowledge on the dentist's part. Evidence-based studies have shown that necessary dental procedures can be performed during the second trimes-ter of pregnancy without an increased risk for serious medical adverse events, spontaneous abortions, preterm deliveries, and fetal mal-formations. The conservative approach of discouraging treatment because of lack of knowledge about the effects of a procedure and/or medication is not typically erring on

Dental Management of the Pregnant Patient, First Edition. Edited by Christos A. Skouteris.
© 2018 John Wiley & Sons, Inc. Published 2018 by John Wiley & Sons, Inc.

Box 1.1 Ethics in the dental management of the pregnant patient.

Applicable principles of the ADA Code of Ethics
- Principle I: Autonomy, Involvement
- Principle II: Nonmaleficence
- Principle IV: Justice
- Principle V: Veracity

---

the side of fetal safety; rather, it suggests a lack of knowledge about whether it is riskier for the fetus to be exposed to a medication or to the effects of untreated maternal morbidity. According to Lyerly *et al.* (2008), in the absence of information about the safety and efficacy of medications, pregnant women and their healthcare providers are left with two unsavory options: take a drug, with unknown safety and efficacy, or fail to treat the condition, thus leaving the woman and fetus vulnerable to the consequences of the underlying medical problems.

Under the principle of **Justice** ("fairness"), a "dentist has a duty to treat people fairly." Moreover, "the dentist's primary obligations include dealing with people justly and delivering dental care without prejudice" and "dentists shall not refuse to accept patients

into their practice or deny dental service to patients because of the patient's sex." Refusing to treat a pregnant patient could be interpreted as discriminating against her unjustly and thus disregarding the ADA Code.

The **Veracity** principle ("truthfulness") refers to the dentist's primary obligations which include respecting the position of trust inherent in the dentist–patient relationship, communicating truthfully and without deception, and maintaining intellectual integrity. The dentist is not truthful if denying treatment to a pregnant patient on the grounds of potential harm to the mother and fetus, when scientific evidence does not support that the pregnancy and the fetus are at risk.

The most serious ethical issues arise in cases of life-threatening conditions, such as head and neck infections, severe maxillofacial trauma, and locally aggressive benign and malignant tumors. These conditions will be discussed later in the book. Under those circumstances, treatment decisions for a pregnant patient necessitate a choice between saving her life and that of the fetus, or other dramatic trade-offs. In such cases, Puls *et al.* (1997) stated that there is general consensus (especially in the wake of the Angela Carder case; Box 1.2) that the primary consideration

---

Box 1.2 The Angela Carder case.

Angela Carder (née Stoner) was diagnosed with Ewing's sarcoma at the age of 13 years. Her prognosis was dismal but following chemotherapy and radiation, she managed to survive and remained in remission for several years. She got married and with her doctors' approval she became pregnant.

In 1987, in her first week of the third trimester of pregnancy, she was found to have recurrence of her disease with lung metastases. She had already fought hard to survive and she requested to be treated again with chemotherapy and radiation which had contributed to her years in remission, in spite of the risks

to the fetus. She was admitted to George Washington University Hospital, in Washington DC, where she was deemed a terminal case. As a result of her condition, there was disagreement as to whether she should be treated, exercising her right to save or prolong her life, at the expense of the life of the fetus. Although her condition deteriorated and she was running out of time, Angela did not elect to have an emergent C-section.

This caused concern among the hospital risk managers who, fearing a lawsuit from pro-life organizations, requested a court hearing on the issue, providing legal representation for

Angela, the fetus, and the hospital. At the hearing, her family and her attending physicians all testified against performing a C-section, based on low survivability for the patient and her expressed desire not to go through with the procedure. Angela was not able to testify during the hearing because of her very poor physical condition. The testimony that tipped the balance in favor of an emergent C-section was that of a neonatologist, not familiar with her condition, who testified that the fetal survival rate was 60%. Interestingly, the same fetal survival rate applies also to pregnant women in good health who are at the same gestational age. Angela's attending oncologist was not asked to testify, although he had expressed the view that the procedure was inadvisable for the patient and the fetus.

The court eventually issued an order for an emergent C-section to be performed, although Angela strenuously objected to it. Only one of the hospital's obstetricians reluctantly agreed to perform the procedure without an informed consent and against the will of the patient. Following the C-section, the fetus is purported to have survived for 2 hours. Angela endured the procedure, was informed about the fate of the fetus, and died 2 days later.

Eventually, in April of 1990 after a legal battle, the US Appellate Court ruled that all previous decisions be annulled and that Angela Carder had the right to make her own decisions relative to her health and the health of her fetus. It was the first Appellate Court decision to take a stand against forced C-sections. The case stands as a landmark in United States case law establishing the rights of pregnant women to determine their own healthcare.

Adapted from Thornton and Paltrow (1991).

should be saving the life of the mother. Charles Weijer (1998) points out, however, that in some cases a pregnant patient's decision to refuse treatment and sacrifice herself for her child should be counted as an autonomous decision worth respecting, and that it should not be assumed that only self-interest decisions can be autonomous.

References

Lyerly AD, Little MO, and Faden RR. (2008) A critique of the fetus as patient. *American Journal of Bioethics*, **8**, 42.

Puls L, Terry R, and Hunter J. (1997) Primary vaginal cancer in pregnancy: difficulty in the ethical management. *Ethics and Medicine*, **13**, 56.

Raimann T. (2016) The ethics of dental treatment during pregnancy. *Journal of the American Dental Association*, **147**, 689.

Thornton TE and Paltrow L (1991) The rights of pregnant patients. Carder case brings bold policy initiatives. *HealthSpan*, **8**(5), 10–16.

Weijer C. (1998) Commentary: self-interest is not the sole legitimate basis for making decisions. *British Medical Journal*, **316**, 850.

Further Reading

Flyn TR and Susarla SM. (2007) Oral and maxillofacial surgery for the pregnant patient. *Oral and Maxillofacial Surgical Clinics of North America*, **19**, 207.

Zalta EN, Nodelman U, Allen C, *et al.* (2011) Pregnancy, birth, and medicine. Stanford Encyclopedia of Philosophy. Available online at: https://plato.stanford.edu/entries/ethics-pregnancy/ (accessed 15 October 2017).

2

Physiologic Changes and Their Sequelae in Pregnancy

Christos A. Skouteris

The physiologic changes that occur during pregnancy are hormonal as well as anatomic, consequently affecting many organs and systems of the female body. These changes can occasionally present as subtle homeostatic alterations that can progress to serious, even life-threatening situations, if they are not recognized early and preventive and management actions are not employed in a timely manner. Pregnancy induces cardiovascular, respiratory, hematologic, urinary, gastrointestinal, hepatobiliary, endocrine, immunologic, dermatologic, musculoskeletal, and psychologic changes that are more dramatic in multifetal than in single pregnancies. Most of these changes return to normal after delivery.

Cardiovascular

The cardiovascular system's response to pregnancy is a dynamic process aiming at providing uteroplacental circulation for normal fetal growth and development. Changes in cardiovascular physiology involve the peripheral vascular resistance, cardiac output, heart rate, stroke volume, and blood pressure (Box 2.1).

Peripheral vascular resistance decreases by approximately 35–40% as a result of systemic vasodilation. Vasodilation is mostly the result of the action of increased concentrations of relaxin, progesterone, and estradiol. Relaxin is a peptide hormone produced by the corpus luteum of the ovary, the breast and, during pregnancy, also by the placenta, chorion, and decidua. This hormone has been shown to have an endothelium-dependent vasodilatory role in pregnancy that can influence small arterial vessel resistance, thus causing an increase in arterial compliance. Nitric oxide was also thought to contribute to the decrease in peripheral vascular resistance through vasodilation, as studies of human hand flow suggested, but studies of forearm flow showed that it does not. The decrease in peripheral resistance starts in the first trimester, is more profound in the second trimester, with a slight upswing during the third trimester of pregnancy.

Cardiac output increases sharply in the first trimester, continues to increase into the second trimester and by the 24th week of gestation has reached a level of 30–50% above the baseline. There is no consensus as to whether any changes in cardiac output occur in the third trimester of pregnancy. The increase in cardiac output in early pregnancy is credited to increased stroke volume whereas the increase in cardiac output in late pregnancy is attributed to the increase in heart rate. Cardiac output falls to nonpregnant values in a few weeks after delivery. The physiologic increase in cardiac output is a compensatory mechanism to counteract the decreased oxygen capacity of maternal blood. Any event from any source that can cause a drop in cardiac output may result in maternal hypoxia and compromise the condition of the fetus.

Dental Management of the Pregnant Patient, First Edition. Edited by Christos A. Skouteris.
© 2018 John Wiley & Sons, Inc. Published 2018 by John Wiley & Sons, Inc.

<table>
<tr><td>

Box 2.1 Most significant cardiovascular changes in pregnancy.

• Peripheral vascular resistance decreases
• Cardiac output increases
• Heart rate increases
• Stroke volume increases
• Blood pressure decreases

</td></tr>
</table>

Heart rate shows a progressive increase by 10–20 bpm during the first and second trimester with a peak in the third trimester. The overall increase in heart rate raises 10–20% above the baseline and remains increased for 2–5 days after delivery.

Stroke volume starts increasing from the eighth week and reaches a peak by the 20th week of pregnancy. It drops back to baseline by the second week post partum. Stroke volume is augmented by the increase in end-diastolic volume and maintenance of ejection fraction through a possible increase in contractile force. The increase is the result of dramatic heart and vascular remodeling during the first few weeks of pregnancy. Heart remodeling is expressed throughout pregnancy by a left ventricular wall thickness and left ventricular wall mass increase by 28% and 52% above pre-pregnancy values respectively, and by a 40% increase in right ventricular mass. Vascular remodeling is demonstrated by an increase in arterial compliance. A measure of increase in arterial compliance is provided by the aortic augmentation index, a marker of aortic stiffness, which decreases significantly early during pregnancy, reaching a lowest point in the second trimester and gradually increasing in the third trimester.

Blood pressure is decreased during pregnancy, including systolic blood pressure, diastolic blood pressure, mean arterial pressure, and central systolic blood pressure. Diastolic blood pressure and mean arterial pressure decrease more than systolic blood pressure. Arterial pressures decrease to a lowest point during the second trimester (dropping 5–10 mmHg below baseline), but the majority of the decrease occurs early

in pregnancy (6–8-week gestational age) compared with nonpregnancy values. This decrease in blood pressure during pregnancy is ascribed to vasodilation mainly caused by relaxin, progesterone, estradiol, prostacyclin, and potentially by nitric oxide.

Respiratory

Respiratory changes affect the condition of the upper airway tissues as much as the pulmonary and respiratory physiology (Boxes 2.2, 2.3). The upper airway undergoes significant mucosal changes. The mucosa becomes friable and edematous. Capillary engorgement causes hyperemia of the nasal and oropharyngeal mucosa and larynx which begins early in the first trimester and increases progressively throughout pregnancy.

<table>
<tr><td>

Box 2.2 Respiratory changes in pregnancy: mucosal/anatomic.

• Upper airway mucosa friable, edematous
• Thoracic cage expands
• Ribs flare
• Diaphragm elevated
• Intrathoracic pressure increases

</td></tr>
</table>

<table>
<tr><td>

Box 2.3 Respiratory changes in pregnancy: Pulmonary/respiratory.

• Respiratory rate unchanged
• Tidal volume increased
• Minute ventilation increased
• Total lung volume decreases
• Vital capacity unchanged
• Residual volume decreased
• Inspiratory reserve volume unchanged
• Expiratory reserve volume decreased
• Forced expiratory volume 1 and ratio to forced vital capacity unchanged
• Maternal/fetal O_2 consumption increased
• Functional residual capacity decreased
• Hyperventilation
• Compensatory respiratory alkalosis
• Dyspnea

</td></tr>
</table>

Respiratory changes in pregnancy: glossary of terms.

- **Tidal volume** (TV): amount of air moving into lungs with each inspiration
- **Inspiratory reserve volume** (IRV): air inspired with maximal inspiratory effort in excess of tidal volume
- **Expiratory reserve volume** (ERV): volume expelled by active expiratory effort after passive expiration
- **Residual volume** (RV): air left in lungs after maximal expiratory effort
- **Vital capacity (VC)**: greater amount of air that can be expired after maximal inspiratory effort
- **Forced vital capacity** (FVC): the amount of air which can be forcibly exhaled after taking the deepest breath possible
- **Minute ventilation** (MV): the total lung ventilation per minute
- **Functional residual capacity** (FRC): volume of air present in the lungs at the end of passive expiration
- **Forced expiratory volume 1**(FEV1): the maximum amount of air expired in 1 second
- **FEV1/FVC ratio**: the proportion of vital capacity that can be expired in the first second of forced expiration

---

Up to one-third of pregnant women experience severe rhinitis, which predisposes them to frequent episodes of epistaxis and upper respiratory tract infections. Polyposis of nose and sinuses may occur and regress after delivery. Airway conductance increases, indicating dilation of the respiratory tract below the larynx. This is mainly due to direct effects of progesterone, cortisone, and relaxin. Another potential mechanism is through enhanced beta-adrenergic activity induced by progesterone.

Anatomic and respiratory compensatory changes are commensurate with the increased oxygen demands of the mother and fetus and are mediated by biochemical and mechanical factors. These changes accommodate the progressive increase in oxygen consumption and the physical impact of the enlarging uterus. Normal oxygen consumption is 250 mL/min at rest and increases by 20% over the nonpregnant state in order to meet the 15% increase in the maternal metabolic rate.

As part of the anatomic adaptations to address these demands, the configuration of the thoracic cage changes early in pregnancy. The shape of the chest changes as diameters increase, by about 2 cm, resulting in a 5–7 cm expansion of the chest circumference. The flaring of the lower ribs causes the diaphragm to rise by up to 4 cm, its contribution to the respiratory effort increasing with no evidence of being impeded by the uterus. These changes are thought to be mediated by the effect of progesterone, which together with relaxin increases ribcage elasticity by relaxing ligaments. Flaring of the ribs results in an increase in the subcostal angle, transverse diameter, and chest circumference. As gestation advances, upward displacement of the diaphragm causes a total lung volume decrease of 5%.

In general, what remains unchanged in the respiratory physiology of the pregnant patient is the respiratory rate, vital capacity (VC), inspiratory reserve volume (IRV), FEV1 or the ratio of FEV1 to forced vital capacity, and the arterial pH.

Gas exchange undergoes significant changes during pregnancy. Tidal volume (TV) and minute ventilation increase by 30–40%. Minute ventilation is increased (primarily an increase in tidal volume with a normal respiratory rate) for two reasons. First, oxygen consumption and carbon dioxide production increase 20–30% by the third trimester and up to 100% during labor, necessitating increased minute ventilation to maintain normal acid–base status. In addition, progesterone directly stimulates the central respiratory center, causing a further increase in minute ventilation. Expiratory reserve volume (ERV), residual volume (RV), and functional residual capacity (FRC) decrease by 20%. The decrease in FRC reaches 80% of nonpregnant value by term. The FRC reduction is further affected by obesity and postural changes. A pregnant woman in the supine position has an FRC 70% of that in the sitting position.

All of these changes in pregnancy result in overcompensation in an effort to meet the maternal and fetal respiratory demands. The resulting *hyperventilation* causes an increase in arterial oxygen tension (PaO_2) and a decrease in arterial carbon dioxide tension ($PaCO_2$). Hyperventilation also seems to be related to an increase in the sensitivity of brainstem respiratory centers to the combined action of $PaCO_2$ and progesterone. The net effect is a mild respiratory alkalosis caused by a compensatory fall in serum bicarbonate (HCO_3-) through an increase of bicarbonate excretion via the kidneys.

Hyperventilation and elevation of the diaphragm are the most likely causes of the so-called *physiologic dyspnea of pregnancy* which is a common complaint of 60–70% of pregnant women. It usually starts late in the first trimester, shows an increased frequency in the second trimester, and remains stable during the third trimester of pregnancy. The mechanism of dyspnea during normal pregnancy is not entirely clear. It occurs while the uterus is still relatively small, so it cannot be attributed solely to an increase in abdominal girth. Hyperventilation is likely to be at least partially responsible, perhaps due to the increase in ventilation above the level needed to meet the rise in metabolic demand. The presence of dyspnea during pregnancy has been found to correlate with a low $PaCO_2$ and the women most likely to experience dyspnea are those who had relatively high baseline nonpregnant values for $PaCO_2$. Although dyspnea in pregnancy is not usually associated with pathologic processes, care must be taken not to dismiss it lightly and miss a warning sign of cardiac or pulmonary disease.

Hematologic

There are a number of profound physiologic hematologic changes that result during normal pregnancy. Some of these, in addition to their clinical implications, can induce significant alterations in laboratory values that in a nonpregnant woman would be considered distinctly abnormal. The most significant hematologic changes are summarized in Box 2.4.

Plasma volume increases 45% at term as a result of the combined action of the renin-angiotensin and aldosterone systems which promote an increase in fluid retention. Plasma volume increases progressively throughout normal pregnancy. Most of this increase occurs by the 34th week of gestation. Plasma volume expansion is required to address the increased maternal-fetal-placental circulatory demands. The red blood cell volume, however, does not show significant change. The net result is a dilutional anemia (physiologic anemia of pregnancy) and a decrease in the serum colloid osmotic pressure. (Figure 2.1, Table 2.1). The physiologic anemia of pregnancy starts in the first trimester, becoming more profound in the third trimester.

Leukocytosis, occurring during pregnancy, is due to the physiologic stress induced by the pregnant state. Neutrophils are the major type of leukocytes on differential counts. This is likely due to impaired neutrophilic apoptosis in pregnancy and as a result of the action of elevated estrogen and cortisol levels. Leukocytosis remains present throughout gestation (Table 2.2).

Box 2.4 Most significant hematologic changes in pregnancy.

- Physiologic anemia
- Leukocytosis (neutrophilia)
- Gestational thrombocytopenia
- Hypercoagulability
- Decreased fibrinolysis

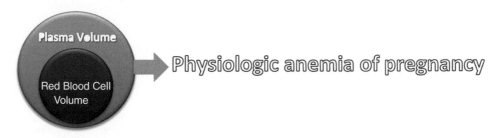

Figure 2.1 Physiologic anemia of pregnancy.

Table 2.1 Hemoglobin/hematocrit range includes references with and without iron supplementation.

	Nonpregnant	First trimester	Second trimester	Third trimester
Hemoglobin (g/dL)	12.0–15.8	11.6–13.9	9.7–14.8	9.5–15.0
Hematocrit (%)	35.4–44.4	31.0–41.0	30.0–39.0	28.0–40.0

Table 2.2 White blood cell and neutrophil count per trimester compared to the nonpregnant status ($\times 10^3/mm^3$).

	Nonpregnant	First trimester	Second trimester	Third trimester
White blood cell count	3.5–9.1	5.7–13.6	5.6–14.8	5.9–16.9
Neutrophils	1.4–4.6	3.6–10.1	3.8–12.3	3.9–13.1

Gestational thrombocytopenia occurs in approximately 8% of all pregnancies and accounts for more than 70% of cases with thrombocytopenia in pregnancy. The pathophysiology is unknown, but certain factors appear to contribute to its manifestation. These include hemodilution, increased platelet consumption, increased platelet aggregation driven by increased levels of thromboxane A2, as well as accelerated platelet activation potentially occurring at placental circulation. (Table 2.3).

Gestational thrombocytopenia is self-limiting, resolves within 1–2 months after delivery, and is not associated with adverse outcomes for the baby.

Hypercoagulability and decreased fibrinolysis are the most important hematologic changes in pregnancy. Although these physiologic changes may be important for minimizing intrapartum blood loss, they entail an increased risk of thromboembolism during pregnancy and the postpartum period. Pregnant women are in a hypercoagulable state throughout gestation due to increased protein synthesis mediated by the rising estrogen levels. Levels of clotting factor and natural anticoagulants undergo significant changes as gestation progresses (Table 2.4).

Systemic fibrinolytic activity is markedly depressed during pregnancy. The decreased fibrinolytic activity is presumed to be caused by loss of plasminogen activator. Recent studies in vitro have shown that antiphospholipid antibodies (aPLs) may interfere with the intrinsic fibrinolysis system. However, the capacity for localized fibrinolytic activity is not lost, because the concentrations of fibrin degradation products and particularly D-Dimer are raised during pregnancy. The overall pattern is one of increased coagulant and reduced fibrinolytic capacity during pregnancy which may protect the pregnant woman against the challenge of placental separation.

Table 2.3 Platelet count per trimester compared to the nonpregnant status ($\times 10^9$/L).

	Nonpregnant	First trimester	Second trimester	Third trimester
Platelets	165–415	174–391	155–409	146–429

Table 2.4 Clotting factor changes.

Clotting factor	Level change during pregnancy
I (fibrinogen)	Increased
II (prothrombin)	Increased
VII (stable factor, proconvertin)	Increased
VIII (antihemophilic factor A)	Increased
IX (antihemophilic factor B or Christmas factor)	Increased
X (Stuart-Prower factor)	Increased
XI (plasma thromboplastin antecedent)	Increased
XII (Hageman factor)	Decreased
XIII (fibrin stabilizing factor)	Decreased
Protein S	Decreased
Protein C	Unchanged
Antithrombin III	Unchanged
Plasminogen	Increased
D-Dimer	Increased

Gastrointestinal

Pregnancy causes anatomic and physiologic changes in the gastrointestinal (GI) tract, which are associated with symptoms of nausea, vomiting, and pyrosis (heartburn) that are the most common complaints in pregnancy (Box 2.5).

Nausea and vomiting are experienced by 50% of women early in their pregnancy. An additional 25% have nausea as the only symptom. The onset of nausea is within 4 weeks after the last menstrual period in most patients. The problem typically peaks at approximately 9 weeks of gestation. Sixty percent of cases resolve by the end of the first trimester, and 91% resolve by 20 weeks of gestation. Nausea and vomiting are less common in older women, multiparous women, and smokers; this observation has been attributed to the smaller placental volumes in these women. Severe, persistent nausea and vomiting in pregnancy, known as *hyperemesis gravidarum*, tends to occur in the first trimester of pregnancy and lasts significantly longer. It is a serious condition that can lead to severe physical and emotional stress, weight loss, dehydration, ketosis, vitamin B1, B6, and B12 deficiency, ketoacidosis, and hyperthyroidism.

Although the cause of nausea and vomiting in pregnancy is unclear, several theories have been proposed to explain the pathophysiology of these symptoms (Box 2.6).

Human chorionic gonadotropin (hCG) is believed to indirectly cause nausea and vomiting in pregnancy through stimulation of ovarian estrogen production that is known to increase nausea and vomiting. This is evidenced by the observation that women with twin pregnancies or with a complete

---

Box 2.5 Most common astrointestinal symptoms in pregnancy.

- Nausea
- Vomiting
- Pyrosis (heartburn)

Box 2.6 Causes of nausea and vomiting in pregnancy.

- Human chorionic gonadotropin (hCG)
- *Helicobacter pylori* (*H. pylori*)
- Vitamin B deficiency
- Gestational trophoblastic disease
- Psychologic – depression
- Cannabinoid hyperemesis syndrome

hydatidiform mole (no fetus), who have higher hCG levels than do other pregnant women, experience clinically significant nausea and vomiting. This also indicates that the stimulus is produced by the placenta and not the fetus.

Helicobacter pylori (*H. pylori*) infection shows an increased incidence in pregnant women. Several studies have shown an association between *H. pylori* infection and the pathophysiology of hyperemesis gravidarum. Contributing factors to the increased incidence may include steroid hormone-induced changes in gastric pH and/or increased susceptibility due to changes in humoral and cell-mediated immunity. *Vitamin B deficiency* may contribute to these symptoms, since the use of multivitamins containing vitamin B reduces the incidence of nausea and vomiting.

Gestational trophoblastic disease, which encompasses a group of rare, pregnancy-related tumors (hydatidiform mole, invasive mole, choriocarcinoma, placental site trophoblastic tumor, and epithelioid trophoblastic tumor), has been implicated in the incidence of nausea and vomiting. These tumors, that develop in the placenta and arise from trophoblastic cells, produce high levels of hCG and particularly of beta-hCG that act through stimulation of estrogen production, as already mentioned.

Psychologic factors such as depression have been suggested as causing nausea and vomiting but there are not enough data in support of potential psychologic connection.

An additional cause of persistent nausea and vomiting is the so-called *cannabinoid hyperemesis syndrome*, which occurs by an unknown mechanism. This condition should be considered in pregnant women with intractable nausea relieved by frequent hot bathing. In view of the legalization of recreational cannabis, the incidence of this syndrome is expected to rise. By considering this diagnosis, extensive diagnostic testing can be avoided and the correct therapy, abstaining from cannabis use, can be recommended.

Pyrosis (heartburn) in pregnancy is mainly the result of gastroesophageal reflux disease (GERD). Pregnancy alters visceral anatomy and affects the normal motility of the esophagus, stomach, and intestines. Gastroesophageal reflux disease, commonly experienced as pyrosis (heartburn), is reported to affect 40–85% of pregnant women in their third trimester. Mechanical and hormonal factors are involved in the pathophysiology of GERD in pregnancy (Box 2.7).

Decreased esophageal sphincter pressure has been attributed to the combined action of progesterone, ethinylestradiol, and 17-beta estradiol through their relaxation effect on the esophageal sphincter smooth muscle.

Increased abdominal pressure and the enlarging gravid uterus may also contribute to the occurrence of gastroesophageal reflux. The enlarging gravid uterus causes increased intraabdominal pressure, thus compressing the stomach and provoking reflux symptoms. However, this mechanism cannot adequately explain the onset of GERD in early pregnancy when the uterus has not yet attained large dimensions.

Slow gastric emptying is the result of alterations of gastrointestinal motility in pregnancy which can promote GERD. The exact pathophysiology behind these gastrointestinal motility alterations is not yet fully understood but it is believed that they are brought about by pregnancy hormones which may affect normal function of the enteric nerves and muscles, resulting in slower motility throughout the gastrointestinal tract.

As part of the gastrointestinal system, the *liver* undergoes certain adaptations during pregnancy that project as changes in liver function. Liver function test values

---

Box 2.7 Causes of GERD in pregnancy.

- Decreased lower esophageal sphincter pressure
- Increased abdominal pressure
- Slow gastric emptying

Table 2.5 Changes in serum liver function tests during normal pregnancy.

Test	First trimester	Second trimester	Third trimester
Albumin	Decreased	Decreased	Decreased
ALT	WNL or slight change	WNL or slight change	WNL or slight change
AST	WNL or slight change	WNL or slight change	WNL or slight change
Total bilirubin	Decreased	Decreased	Decreased
ALP	WNL or slight change	WNL or increased	Increased
GGT	WNL or slight change	Decreased	Decreased
5'NT	WNL or slight change	WNL or increased	WNL or slight change
TBA (fasting state)	WNL or slight change	WNL or slight change	WNL or slight change
PT	WNL or slight change	WNL or slight change	WNL or slight change

5'NT, 5'-nucleotidase; ALP, alkaline phosphatase; ALT, alanine aminotransferase; AST, aspartate aminotransferase; GGT, gamma-glutamyltransferase; PT, prothrombin time; TBA, total bile acids; WNL, within normal limits in reference to normal nonpregnant women.

compared with nonpregnancy values are representative of these changes (Table 2.5). The physiologic changes in liver function in pregnancy are commonly transient, remain only during pregnancy, and correct spontaneously in the postpartum period.

Caution: Any increase in serum ALT and AST activity levels, serum GGT activity, serum bilirubin or fasting total bile acid concentrations should be considered pathologic, and should prompt further evaluation.

Genitourinary

Pregnancy affects both the kidney and urinary tract anatomy and function with an expression in laboratory values (Boxes 2.8, 2.9).

Kidney size increases by 1–1.5 cm. Vascular and interstitial spaces increase in volume which in turn increases the volume of the kidneys by 30%. Kidney size is also affected by hydroureter and hydronephrosis secondary to dilation of the renal calyces, pelvices, and ureters as a result of progesterone effects and ureteric mechanical obstruction. Up to 80% of pregnant women develop hydroureter and hydronephrosis, more prominent on the

Box 2.8 Anatomic genitourinary changes in pregnancy.

- Kidney size increased
- Renal calyces dilated
- Renal pelvices dilated
- Ureters dilated

Box 2.9 Functional genitourinary changes in pregnancy.

- Renal plasma flow (RPF) increases
- Total body water increases
- Glomerular filtration rate (GFR) increases
- Urinary protein excretion increases
- Glycosuria increases
- Aminoaciduria increases

right side because of the anatomic relation of the ureter with the iliac and ovarian vessels before it enters into the renal pelvis. These changes can be visualized on ultrasound examination by the second trimester, and may not resolve until 6–12 weeks postpartum.

Renal plasma flow (RPF) increases as a result of increased cardiac output and systemic vasodilation.

Total body water increase is the result, at least in part, of the upregulation of renin-angiotensin-aldosterone system (RAAS) activity. One of the stimuli for this increased activity could be systemic vasodilation, leading to a relatively lower volume and pressure state. This leads to retention of about 900–1000 mEq of sodium and a 6–8 L increase in total body water, of which 4–6 L are located in the extracellular compartment.

One of the earliest kidney changes is the impressive rise in *glomerular filtration rate* (GFR). In an elegant study of 11 healthy women, Davison and Noble (1981) documented serial measurements of creatinine clearance using 24-hour urine collections during the menstrual cycle through conception and up to 16 weeks of gestation. GFR rises to a peak of 40–50% that of nonpregnancy levels. As a result of the increased filtration, clearance of creatinine, uric acid, and urea is increased, which results in a decline in serum creatinine, uric acid, and blood urea nitrogen (Table 2.6). GFR increase has been linked to the increase of RPF but this association is not constant throughout pregnancy. Luteal phase progesterone may also play a role in increasing RPF and GFR, and its role may continue during pregnancy.

Urinary protein excretion increases during pregnancy. Both total protein excretion and urinary albumin excretion are increased compared with nonpregnant levels, particularly after 20 weeks of gestation. Increased GFR and possibly urinary tract dilation as well as alterations in glomerular charge selectivity may also contribute to physiologic gestational proteinuria and albuminuria. Based on the results of a longitudinal study evaluating women before conception, through pregnancy, and post partum, as well as on smaller cross-sectional studies, the average 24-hour total protein and albumin excretion is 200 mg and 12 mg, respectively, with upper limits of 300 mg/24 h and 20 mg/24 h. Proteinuria in excess of 300 mg/24 h is pathologic and warrants prompt attention.

Glycosuria occurs in normal pregnancy with a several-fold increase in the amount of glucose excreted in the urine in the third trimester compared with the small amount (<125 mg/day) excreted by nonpregnant individuals. Normally, glucose is freely filtered and almost completely reabsorbed by a sodium-coupled active transport in the proximal tubule. A small amount of glucose is also absorbed in the collecting tubule. In pregnancy, an increase in plasma volume results in both an increased GFR and an increased tubular flow rate. This increased flow rate may limit the ability of the proximal tubule to completely reabsorb glucose, resulting in physiologic glycosuria of pregnancy.

Aminoaciduria is the presence of amino acids in the urine. Small amounts of amino acids occur in the urine of nonpregnant women. In pregnancy, there is an increase in fractional excretion of alanine, glycine,

Table 2.6 Average laboratory values in pregnancy.

Laboratory variables	Nonpregnant	First trimester	Second trimester	Third trimester
Plasma osmolality (mOsm/kg H_2O)	275–295	275–280	276–289	278–280
Serum sodium (mEq/L)	136–146	133–148	129–148	130–148
Serum potassium (mEq/L)	3.5–5.0	3.6–5.0	3.3–5.0	3.3–5.1
Serum bicarbonate (mmol/L)	22–30	20–24	20–24	20–24
Serum creatinine (mg/dL)	0.5–0.9	0.4–0.7	0.4–0.8	0.4–0.9
Blood urea nitrogen (mg/dL)	7–20	7–12	3–13	3–11
Uric acid (mg/dL)	2.5–5.6	2.0–4.2	2.4–4.9	3.1–6.3

histidine, serine, and threonine. The mechanism of this selective gestational aminoaciduria remains unknown.

Endocrine

Maternal endocrine adaptations to pregnancy involve the hypothalamus, pituitary, parathyroid, thyroid, adrenal glands, and ovary, and are linked to the interactions of the fetal-placental-maternal unit. Besides the physiologic changes triggered in other organ systems by the estrogens and progesterone, the hormonal role of the placenta is pivotal in activating and regulating endocrine changes during pregnancy. The physiologic endocrine adaptations are anatomic as well as functional (Box 2.10).

The *pituitary* enlarges 2–3-fold during pregnancy. The peak maternal pituitary size may reach 12 mm in the first days post partum, but involutes rapidly thereafter and

---

Box 2.10 Endocrine changes in pregnancy.

Anatomic

- Pituitary size increased
- Thyroid gland size slightly increased
- Parathyroid size increased
- Adrenal size unchanged
- Pancreas size unchanged

Functional

- Pituitary: ACTH, prolactin levels increase
- Growth hormone within normal limits
- Thyroid: TSH decreases
- TBG, total T3, T4 levels* increase
- Parathyroid: PTH stable
- Adrenals: aldosterone and cortisol levels increase
- Pancreas: insulin concentration increases

ACTH, adrenocorticotropic hormone; PTH, parathyroid hormone; TBG, thyroxine-binding globulin; TSH, thyroid-stimulating hormone.
*Free T3 and T4 levels remain unchanged.

---

reaches normal size by 6 months post partum. This enlargement is primarily caused by estrogen-stimulated hypertrophy and hyperplasia of the prolactin-producing cells of the pituitary. Maternal plasma prolactin levels parallel the increase in pituitary size throughout gestation. Pregnancy dramatically affects the hypothalamic-pituitary-adrenal axis, leading to increased circulating cortisol and adrenocorticotropic hormone (ACTH), whereas serum growth hormone (GH) levels measured with the use of a sensitive radioimmunoassay under conditions in which there was minimal interference from placental lactogen (HPL) are within normal limits during gestation.

Thyroid gland vascularity increases and glandular hyperplasia occurs as a result of the increased need for thyroid hormone production, leading to slightly increased size of the thyroid gland during pregnancy. Production of thyroid hormones T3 and T4 increases by about 50%. As a result, the normal thyroid-stimulating hormone (TSH) level during pregnancy is lower than the normal nonpregnancy level. Total T3 and T4 levels increase but do not result in hyperthyroidism because of the parallel increase in thyroxine-binding globulin (TBG).

The size of the *parathyroid glands* increases slightly but maternal parathyroid hormone (PTH) remains stable during pregnancy.

The maternal *adrenal gland* does not change morphologically during pregnancy. Plasma adrenal steroid levels increase with advancing gestation. Plasma and urinary free cortisol increase 2–3 times, but pregnant women normally do not exhibit any overt clinical features of hypercortisolism. Levels of renin and angiotensin rise during pregnancy, leading to elevated angiotensin II levels and markedly elevated levels of aldosterone.

The most important function of the *pancreas* in pregnancy is the regulation of insulin response to nutrients. Fasting plasma insulin increases gradually during pregnancy – by the third trimester levels are two-fold higher than before pregnancy. During normal pregnancy, oral and intravenous glucose tolerance deteriorates only slightly, despite the reduction in insulin sensitivity. The main mechanism responsible for that phenomenon is a gradual increase in insulin secretion by the beta-cells. The mechanism responsible for increased insulin secretion during pregnancy is not well understood. A major contributing factor is the increase in the beta-cell mass, a combination of hyperplasia and hypertrophy. The increased beta-cell mass can contribute to the increased fasting insulin concentration despite normal or lowered fasting glucose concentrations in late pregnancy, and to the enhanced insulin response to glucose during pregnancy (2–3-fold above nonpregnant levels).

Immunologic

The maternal immune system during pregnancy is altered to actively tolerate the semiallogeneic fetus. These alterations include changes in local immune responses, that is, in the uterine mucosa (decidua), and changes in peripheral immune responses (Box 2.11). Both cell-mediated and humoral immunity show gestational adaptations compared to nonpregnancy status.

Although progesterone seems to have immunosuppressive properties, the concept that pregnancy is associated with immune suppression is not supported by medical and evolutionary evidence. The maternal-fetal-placental axis provides an active immune system that will modify the way the mother responds to the environment. Therefore, it is appropriate to refer to pregnancy as a unique

---

Box 2.11 Immunologic changes in pregnancy.

- Macrophages increased
- Neutrophils increased
- Immature dendritic cells (iDC) decreased
- Natural killer cells (NK) decreased
- Regulatory T cells (Treg) increased

---

immune condition that is modulated, but not suppressed. The role of this immunologic modulation in pregnancy is, on one hand, to maintain pregnancy by creating a transient tolerant microenvironment within the maternal uterus and, on the other hand, to protect the mother and fetus from infections. Immature dendritic cells (iDC), natural killer cells (NK), and regulatory T cells (Treg) are of particular importance for pregnancy maintenance and maternal immunologic tolerance by preventing rejection of the fetus. Cell-mediated and humoral immunity have a crucial role in maternal and fetal protection from viruses and other pathogens.

Cell-Mediated Immunity

Cell-mediated immunity involves lymphocyte recognition of intracellular pathogens, followed by destruction of the infected host cells. The distinction between cell-mediated and humoral immunity lies in the fact that in cell-mediated immunity, the immune response is stimulated by T-helper type I (Th1) lymphocytes and Th1-associated cytokines. Cytotoxic T lymphocytes are the main immune cells that recognize foreign antigens on the surface of infected cells as well as viruses and other intracellular pathogens. The cell-mediated immune response is critical for controlling such pathogens because their intracellular location shelters them from antibody binding.

Humoral Immunity

Humoral or antibody-mediated immunity is triggered by specific antibody pathogen recognition. Humoral immunity is most effective against extracellular pathogens and has a pivotal role in fighting many bacterial infections. Antibody-coated bacteria mediate the uptake of pathogens by phagocytic cells, including neutrophils and macrophages. Bacterial antigens present on the surface of the macrophages stimulate B lymphocytes specific to the pathogen, with ensuing increased B cell production of antibodies to control the infection. This humoral immune response is augmented by T-helper type II (Th2) lymphocytes, which also stimulate and induce B cell replication. The Th2 response during pregnancy results in vigorous anti-body-mediated immunity to pathogens.

Irrespective of the maternal immune response modulation, most pregnant women experience a healthy pregnancy, suggesting that the immunologic changes do not dramatically affect the integrity of the mother. However, it has been shown that pregnant women are more sensitive to certain infections. For instance, the risk of developing clinical disease after infection with poliovirus or hepatitis A virus is increased in pregnant women. Pregnancy has also been shown to increase the possibility of cytomegalovirus, herpes simplex virus, and malaria infection. Maternal immune responses are also reflected by changes in autoimmune diseases. Rheumatoid arthritis often improves during pregnancy, while systemic lupus erythematosus can show an upsurge. However, pregnancy should not imply greater susceptibility to infectious diseases; instead, there is a modulation of the immune system which leads to different responses depending not only on the microorganisms but also on the stages of pregnancy.

Dermatologic

The maternal hormonal status precipitates many physiologic skin changes. Although normal during pregnancy, they may cause considerable patient discomfort and apprehension but should not be confused with true skin diseases (Box 2.12).

Hyperpigmentation in pregnancy is mainly manifest in the form of the linea nigra (a dark line that runs vertically along the midline of the abdomen from the pubis to the umbilicus), darkening of the areolae, melasma, also known as chloasma or mask of pregnancy (dark, irregular, well-demarcated hyperpigmented macules to patches commonly found on the upper cheek, nose, lips, and forehead),

Box 2.12 Physiologic skin changes in pregnancy.

- Hyperpigmentation
- Melasma
- Striae distensae
- Pruritus gravidarum
- Hair and nail changes
- Vascular changes
- Eccrine/apocrine gland activity

darkening and increase in size of existing nevi (it is common for nevi on the breasts and abdomen to grow with normal skin expansion, but recent studies suggest that pregnancy does not induce significant physiologic changes in nevi), and vulvar melanosis (intensely pigmented irregular macules, clinically mimicking malignant melanoma, appearing on the vulva).

Striae distensae (stretch marks) appear as pink-purple, atrophic lines or bands on the abdomen, buttocks, breasts, thighs, or arms. The cause of striae is multifactorial and includes physical factors (e.g., actual stretching of the skin) and hormonal factors (e.g., effects of adrenocortical steroids, estrogen, and relaxin on the skin's elastic fibers). Striae gravidarum occur in up to 90% of pregnant women by the third trimester.

Pruritus gravidarum affects one in five pregnant women and presents as severe pruritus without associated rash, secondary to intrahepatic cholestasis and bile salt retention that is thought to be caused by estrogens and environmental as well as nutritional factors. Jaundice may be present, accounting for approximately 20% of cases of jaundice in pregnancy. Usually occurs during late second (20%) and third trimester (80%) and peaks in the last month before delivery. The palms and soles are frequently affected and, when generalized, it is associated with secondary skin excoriations.

Hair changes occur during pregnancy in the form of hirsutism (on the face, limbs, and back caused by endocrine changes) and post partum with a condition known as *telogen effluvium*. It is characterized by excessive shedding of hair that occurs 1–5 months following pregnancy. This condition is not uncommon, as it affects 40–50% of women. However, like most changes during pregnancy, it limits itself and resolves after a period of 3–6 months.

Nail changes during pregnancy present clinically as increased brittleness, transverse grooves, distal onycholysis (spontaneous separation of the nail plate starting at the distal free margin and progressing proximally), longitudinal melanonychia (a black or brown pigmentation of the normal nail plate), and subungual hyperkeratosis (scaling under the nail due to excessive proliferation of keratinocytes in the nail bed and hyponychium).

Vascular changes in pregnancy are associated with spider telangectasias, palmar erythema, saphenous varicosities, vulvar and hemorrhoidal varicosities, edema (face, eyelids, and extremities), vaginal erythema (Chadwick's sign), and a bluish discoloration of the cervix (Goodell's sign). Vasomotor instability also may cause facial flushing, dermatographism, hot and cold sensations, and marble skin, a condition characterized by bluish skin discoloration from an exaggerated response to cold.

Eccrine gland activity is increased (hyperhidrosis), possibly because of an increase in thyroid activity, whereas *apocrine gland* activity is reduced (hypohidrosis and decreased apocrine secretion), possibly as a result of hormonal changes. Sebaceous gland activity is increased (third trimester) due to increased ovarian and placental androgens, causing what most pregnant women refer to as "greasy skin."

Musculoskeletal

During the later stages of pregnancy weight gain, hormonal changes, and biomechanical adaptations cause considerable functional stress on the axial skeleton and pelvis. Consequently, the musculoskeletal system is affected in a variety of ways.

- Force across some joints is increased up to two-fold.
- Lower back lordosis, flexion of the neck, and shoulder drop change the center of gravity to counterbalance uterus enlargement.
- Abdominal muscles stretch, weaken, and separate, disturbing neutral posture and placing paraspinal muscles under increased tension.
- The width and mobility of the sacroiliac joints and pubic symphysis increase to accommodate the passage of the fetus during labor.
- The anterior tilt of the pelvis is increased significantly with concomitant increase in the use of the hip extensor, abductor, and ankle plantar flexor muscles.

The changes in body habitus and center of gravity may lead to a transient decrease of coordination and predispose pregnant women to minor trauma, such as contusions and bruising, as a result of loss of balance and falls.

Psychologic and Behavioral Changes

Pregnancy is a very important chapter in a woman's life. The changes in maternal physiology have a direct bearing on personality and behavioral patterns during pregnancy and lactation. Psychologic changes and associated behaviors are triggered not only by uterine enlargement and hormone levels, but also by the woman's culture. Sjogren *et al.* (2000), using the Karolinska Scales of Personality (KSP), studied 15 subsets of the scale in 200 women in early and late pregnancy and at 3 and 6 months after delivery. The subsets included:

- Somatic Anxiety
- Muscular Tension
- Psychic Anxiety
- Psychasthenia
- Inhibition of Aggression
- Impulsiveness
- Monotony Avoidance

- Socialization
- Detachment
- Social Desirability
- Indirect Aggression
- Verbal Aggression
- Irritability
- Suspicion
- Guilt.

The authors concluded that:

> "Although most personality traits are stable during the first pregnancy and lactation, some important changes occur toward a lifestyle characterized by less anxiety, more calmness and tolerance for monotony and increased social interaction. These adaptations seem to occur around delivery and the first weeks of lactation and are meaningful for the development of the maternal role. Breastfeeding seemed to promote personality characteristics in this phase of life."

Wiklund *et al.* (2009) studied the changes in maternal personality in relation to the mode of delivery on the basis of the KSP. Their conclusion was that:

> "Personality could be one factor among others influencing women's perceptions of mode of delivery, although personality factors are not protective against operative delivery. It is possible that for some women with high integrity a spontaneous vaginal delivery could be recalled as undignified and frightening. The woman's autonomy in this situation is difficult to ignore because we know that becoming a mother is also sometimes a time of a role conflict because of the diverse responsibilities of the new role."

It has been shown that psychologic and behavioral patterns differ during the trimesters of pregnancy. During the first trimester, pregnant women express excitement about their pregnancy, anger if the pregnancy was not planned and ambivalence about a planned pregnancy. The pregnant woman may also be anxious about her ability to handle the labor and care of the newborn. The second trimester is frequently characterized as a time of psychologic well-being. During this time, a pregnant woman can also be perceived as self-absorbed and introverted. As the pregnancy progresses, the woman may have both positive and negative feelings about the changes in the size and shape of her body. In the third trimester anxiety sets in about the birth; there may be concerns about changes in relationships with a partner, family, and friends, and financial worries. At the same time, the woman may feel excited about the forthcoming birth of her baby and the start of a new phase in her life.

Physiologic changes and their sequelae in pregnancy: take-home message.

Knowledge of the physiologic changes that occur in pregnancy is essential for the proper dental and medical management of the pregnant patient. Erroneous perception of physiologic changes as pathologic, that could result in unnecessary referrals, diagnostic testing, and delay or refusal of treatment, could be detrimental for the well-being of the mother and fetus, particularly when a pregnant patient is in need of emergency, preventive, or restorative treatment. Finally, since the number of pregnancies in women in their late 30s has increased over the past decade, it should be noted that physiologic changes in the various maternal systems may have a different clinical expression in pregnant women of advanced age, mainly because older women are more likely to have preexisting medical conditions.

References

Davison JM, Noble MC. (1981) Serial changes in 24 hour creatinine clearance during normal menstrual cycles and the first trimester of pregnancy. *British*

Journal of Obstetrics and Gynaecology, **88**, 10.

Sjogren B, Widström AM, Edman G, *et al.* (2000) Changes in personality pattern during the first pregnancy and lactation. *Journal of Psychosomatic Obstetrics and Gynecology*, **21**, 31.

Wiklund I, Klundi I, Edman G, *et al.* (2009) First-time mothers and changes in personality in relation to mode of delivery. *Journal of Advanced Nursing*, **65**, 1636.

Further Reading

Abrams ET and Miller EM. (2011) The roles of the immune system in women's reproduction. Evolutionary constraints and life history trade-offs. *American Journal of Physical Anthropology*, **146**, 134.

Airoldi J and Weinstein L. (2007) Clinical significance of proteinuria in pregnancy. *Obstetrics and Gynecology Survey*, **62**, 117.

Ali RAR and Egan LJ. (2007) Gastroesophageal reflux disease in pregnancy. *Best Practice and Research in Clinical Gastroenterology*, **21**, 793.

Alto WA. (2005) No need for glycosuria/proteinuria screen in pregnant women. *Journal of Family Practice*, **54**, 978.

Baeyens L, Hindi S, Sorenson, RL, *et al.* (2016) β-Cell adaptation in pregnancy. *Diabetes, Obesity and Metabolism*, **18**, 63.

Berg G, Hammar M and Moller-Nielsen J. (1988) Low back pain during pregnancy. *Obstetrics and Gynecology*, **71**, 71.

Berghout A and Wiersinga W. (1998) Thyroid size and thyroid function during pregnancy. an analysis. *European Journal of Endocrinology*, **138**, 536.

Bernstein IM, Ziegler W, and Badger GJ. (2001) Plasma volume expansion in early pregnancy. *Obstetrics and Gynecology*, **97**, 669.

Bliddal M, Pottegard A, Kirkegaard H, *et al.* (2016) Association of pre-pregnancy body mass index, pregnancy-related weight changes, and parity with the risk of developing degenerative musculoskeletal conditions. *Arthritis and Rheumatism*, **68** (5), 1156–1164.

Bremme KA. (2003) Haemostatic changes in pregnancy. *Best Practice and Research in Clinical Gastroenterology*, **16**, 152.

Chandra S, Tripathi AK, Mishra S, *et al.* (2012) Physiological changes in hematological parameters during pregnancy. *Indian Journal of Hematology and Blood Transfusion*, **28**, 144–146.

Charan M and Katz PO. (2001) Gastroesophageal reflux disease in pregnancy. *Current Treatment Options in Gastroenterology*, **4**, 73.

Chen SJ, Liu YL, and Sytwu HK. (2012) Immunologic regulation in pregnancy. From mechanism to therapeutic strategy for immunomodulation. *Clinical and Developmental Immunology*, **2012**, 1.

Cheung KL and Lafayette RA. (2013) Renal physiology of pregnancy. *Advances in Chronic Kidney Disease*, **20**, 209.

Chung E and Leinwand LA. (2014) Pregnancy as a cardiac stress model. *Cardiovascular Research*, **101**, 561.

Cunningham FG. (2010) Laboratory values in normal pregnancy, in Protocols for High-Risk Pregnancies, 5th edn (eds JT Qeenan, JC Hobbins JC, CY Spong), Blackwell Science, Oxford.

Dahlgren J. (2006) Pregnancy and insulin resistance. *Metabolic Syndrome and Related Disorders*, **4**, 149.

Dinç H, Esen F, Demirci A, *et al.* (1998) Pituitary dimensions and volume measurements in pregnancy and post partum. *MR assessment. Acta Radiologica*, **39**, 64.

Ellegård EK. (2003) The etiology and management of pregnancy rhinitis. *American Journal of Respiratory Medicine*, **2**, 469.

Fadel HE, Northrop G, Misenhimer HR, *et al.* (1979) Normal pregnancy. a model of sustained respiratory alkalosis. *Journal of Perinatal Medicine*, **7**, 195.

Feldt-Rasmussen U and Mathiesen ER. (2011) Endocrine disorders in pregnancy. physiological and hormonal aspects of pregnancy. *Best Practice and Research in Clinical Endocrinology and Metabolism*, **25**, 875.

Fernández-Suárez A, Pascual VT, Gimenez MT, *et al.* (2003) Immature granulocyte detection by the SE-9000 haematology analyser during pregnancy. *Clinical and Laboratory Hematology*, **25**, 347.

Fowden AL, Sferruzzi-Perri AN, Coan PM, *et al.* (2009) Placental efficiency and adaptation. *Endocrine regulation. Journal of Physiology*, **587**, 3459.

Galli JA, Sawaya RA, and Friedenberg FK. (2011) Cannabinoid hyperemesis syndrome. *Current Drug Abuse Reviews*, **4**, 241.

Gilroy RJ, Mangura BT, and Lavietes MH. (1988) Rib cage and abdominal volume displacements during breathing in pregnancy. *American Review of Respiratory Disease*, **137**, 668.

Golberg D, Szilagyi A, and Graves L. (2007) Hyperemesis gravidarum and Helicobacter pylori infection. A systemic review. *Obstetrics and Gynecology*, **110**, 695.

Goldsmith LT and Weiss G. (2009) Relaxin in human pregnancy. *Annals of the New York Academy of Science*, **1160**, 130.

Grindheim G, Estensen ME, Langesaeter E, *et al.* (2011) Changes in blood pressure during healthy pregnancy. a longitudinal cohort study. *Journal of Hypertension*, **30**, 342.

Grindheim G, Toska K, Estensen ME, *et al.* (2012) Changes in pulmonary function during pregnancy: a longitudinal cohort study. *British Journal of Obstetrics and Gynaecology*, **119**, 94.

Hall ME, George EM, and Grangerb JP. (2011) The heart during pregnancy. *Revista Espagnola de Cardiologia*, **64**, 1045.

Hauguel-de Mouzon S and Lassance L. (2015) Endocrine and metabolic adaptations to pregnancy: impact of obesity. *Hormone Molecular Biology and Clinical Investigation*, **24**, 65.

Hegewald MJ and Crapo RO. (2011) Respiratory physiology in pregnancy. *Clinics in Chest Medicine*, **32**, 1.

Hershman JM. (1999) Human chorionic gonadotropin and the thyroid. Hyperemesis gravidarum and trophoblastic tumors. *Thyroid*, **9**, 653.

Higby K, Suiter CR, Phelps JY, *et al.* (1994) Normal values of urinary albumin and total protein excretion during pregnancy. *American Journal of Obstetrics and Gynecology*, **171**, 984.

Holmgren K and Uddenberg N. (1993) Ambivalence during early pregnancy among expectant mothers. *Gynecology and Obstetrics Investigation*, **36**, 15.

Howie PW. (1979) Blood clotting and fibrinolysis in pregnancy. *Postgraduate Medical Journal*, **55**, 362.

Hsu P and Nanan RK. (2014) Innate and adaptive immune interactions at the fetal-maternal interface in healthy human pregnancy and pre-eclampsia. *Frontiers of Immunology*, **5**, 125.

Hussein W and Lafayette RA. (2014) Renal function in normal and disordered pregnancy. *Current Opinion in Nephrology and Hypertension*, **23**, 46.

Hytten FE and Cheyne GA. (1972) The aminoaciduria of pregnancy. *British Journal of Obstetrics and Gynaecology*, **79**, 424.

James AH. (2009) Pregnancy-associated thrombosis. *Hematology*, **2009**, 277.

Jamjute P, Ahmad A, Ghosh T, *et al.* (2009) Liver function test and pregnancy. *Journal of Maternal, Fetal and Neonatal Medicine*, **22**, 274.

Jensen D, Duffin J, Lam YM, *et al.* (2008) Physiological mechanisms of hyperventilation during human pregnancy. *Respiratory Physiology and Neurobiology*, **161**, 76.

Jeyabalan A and Lain KY. (2007) Anatomic and functional changes of the upper urinary tract during pregnancy. *Urologic Clinics of North America*, **34**, 1.

Jones SV, Ambros-Rudolph C, and Nelson-Piercy C. (2014) Skin disease in pregnancy. *British Medical Journal*, **348**, 6.

Kocak I, Akcan Y, Ustun C, *et al.* (1999) Helicobacter pylori seropositivity in patients with hyperemesis gravidaum. *International Journal of Gynaecology and Obstetrics*, **66**, 251.

Kolarzyk E, Szot WM, and Lyszczarz J. (2005) Lung function and breathing regulation parameters during pregnancy. *Archives of Gynecology and Obstetrics*, **272**, 53.

Kramer J, Bowen A, Stewart N, *et al.* (2013) Nausea and vomiting of pregnancy. prevalence, severity and relation to psychosocial health. *American Journal of Maternal/Child Nursing*, **38**, 21.

Kühl C. (1991) Insulin secretion and insulin resistance in pregnancy and GDM. Implications for diagnosis and management. *Diabetes*, **40**, 18.

Kurien S, Kattimani VS, Sriram R, *et al.* (2013) Management of pregnant patient in dentistry. *Journal of International Oral Health*, **5**, 88.

Lanciers S, Despinasse B, Mehta DI, *et al.* (1999) Increased susceptibility to Helicobacter pylori infection in pregnancy. *Infectious Diseases in Obstetrics and Gynecology*, **7**, 195.

Leber A, Teles A, and Zenclussen AC. (2010) Regulatory T cells and their role in pregnancy. *American Journal of Reproductive Immunology*, **63**, 445.

Lee NM and Saha S. (2011) Nausea and vomiting of pregnancy. *Gastroenterology Clinics of North America*, **40**, 309.

Lee RV. (2000) Symptoms produced by normal physiologic changes in pregnancy, in Medical Care of the Pregnant Patient (eds RV Lee, K Rosene-Montella, LA Barbour, *et al.*), ACP-ASIM, Philadelphia, pp. 52–67.

Lindsay JR and Nieman LK. (2006) Adrenal disorders in pregnancy. *Endocrinology and Metabolism Clinics of North America*, **35**, 1.

LoMauro A and Aliverti A. (2015) Respiratory physiology of pregnancy. *Breathe*, **11**, 297.

Lønberg U, Damm P, Andersson AM, *et al.* (2003) Increase in maternal placental growth hormone during pregnancy and disappearance during parturition in normal and growth hormone-deficient pregnancies. *American Journal of Obstetrics and Gynecology*, **188**, 247.

Longo LD. (1983) Maternal blood volume and cardiac output during pregnancy. a hypothesis of endocrinologic control. *American Journal of Physiology*, **245**, R720.

Lukaski HC, Siders WA, Nielsen EJ, *et al.* (1994) Total body water in pregnancy. assessment by using bioelectrical impedance. *American Journal of Clinical Nutrition*, **59**, 578.

MacLean MA, Wilson R, Thomson JA, *et al.* (1992) Immunological changes in normal pregnancy. *European Journal of Obstetrics, Gynecology and Reproductive Biology*, **43**, 167.

Maharajan A, Aye C, Ratnavel R, *et al.* (2013) Skin eruptions specific to pregnancy. An overview. *Obstetrician and Gynaecologist*, **15**, 233.

Mahendru AA, Everett TR, Wilkinson IB, *et al.* (2014) A longitudinal study of maternal cardiovascular function from preconception to the postpartum period. *Journal of Hypertension*, **32**, 849.

Mastorakos G and Ilias I. (2000) Maternal hypothalamic-pituitary-adrenal axis in pregnancy and the postpartum period. Postpartum-related disorders. *Annals of the New York Academy of Science*, **900**, 95.

Matthews A, Dowswell T, Haas DM, *et al.* (2010) Interventions for nausea and vomiting in early pregnancy. *Cochrane Database of Systematic Reviews*, **9**, CD007575.

Matthews JH, Benjamin S, Gill DS, *et al.* (1990) Pregnancy-associated thrombocytopenia. definition, incidence and natural history. *Acta Haematologica*, **84**, 24.

Maul H, Longo M, Saade GR, *et al.* (2003) Nitric oxide and its role during pregnancy. From ovulation to delivery. *Current Pharmaceutical Design*, **9**, 3590.

Maynard SE and Thadhani R. (2009) Pregnancy and the kidney. *Journal of the American Society of Nephrology*, **20**, 14.

Meah VL, Cockcroft JR, Backx K, *et al.* (2016) Cardiac output and related haemodynamics during pregnancy: a series of meta-analyses. *Heart*, **102**, 490.

Minakami H, Kuwata T, and Sato I. (1996) Gestational thrombocytopenia: is it new? *American Journal of Obstetrics and Gynecology*, **175**, 1676.

Molberg P, Johnson C, and Brown TS. (1994) Leukocytosis in labor: what are its implications? *Family Practice Research Journal*, **14**, 229.

Mor G and Cardenas I. (2010) The immune system in pregnancy. A unique complexity. *American Journal of Reproductive Immunology*, **63**, 425.

Morelli SS, Mandal M, Goldsmith LT, *et al.* (2015) The maternal immune system during pregnancy and its influence on fetal development. *Research and Reports in Biology*, **6**, 171.

Neilson JP. (2008) Interventions for heartburn in pregnancy (review). *Cochrane Database of Systematic Reviews*, **4**, CD007065.

Niebyl JR. (2010) Nausea and vomiting in pregnancy. *New England Journal of Medicine*, **363**, 1544.

Niebyl JR and Goodwin TM. (2002) Overview of nausea and vomiting of pregnancy with an emphasis on vitamins and ginger. *American Journal of Obstetrics and Gynecology*, **186**, 253.

Odutayo A and Hladunewich M. (2012) Obstetric nephrology. Renal hemodynamic and metabolic physiology in normal pregnancy. *Clinical Journal of the American Society of Nephrology*, **7**, 2073.

Olophant SS, Nygaard IE, Zong W, *et al.* (2014) Maternal adaptations in preparation for parturition predict uncomplicated spontaneous delivery outcome. *American Journal of Obstetrics and Gynecology*, **211**, 630.

Page EW and Page EP. (1953) Leg cramps in pregnancy. *Obstetrics and Gynecology*, **1**, 94.

Patterson DA, Smith EL, Monahan M, *et al.* (2010) Cannabinoid hyperemesis and compulsive bathing: a case series and paradoxical pathophysiological explanation. *Journal of the American Board of Family Medicine*, **23**, 790.

Perepu U and Rosenstein L. (2013) Maternal thrombocytopenia in pregnancy. *Proceedings in Obstetrics and Gynecology*, **3**, 6.

Poole JA and Claman HN. (2004) Immunology of pregnancy. Implications for the mother. *Clinical Reviews in Allergy and Immunology*, **26**, 161.

Pramanik SS, Pramanik T, Mondal SC, *et al.* (2007) Number, maturity and phagocytic activity of neutrophils in the three trimesters of pregnancy. *Eastern Mediterranean Health Journal*, **13**, 862.

Racicot K, Kwon JY, Aldo P, *et al.* (2014) Understanding the complexity of the immune system during pregnancy. *American Journal of Reproductive Immunology*, **72**, 107.

Rasmussen PE and Nielsen FR. (1988) Hydronephrosis during pregnancy: a literature survey. *European Journal of Obstetrics, Gynecology and Reproductive Biology*, **27**, 249.

Richter JE. (2005) The management of heartburn in pregnancy. *Alimentary Pharmacology and Therapeutics*, **22**, 749.

Robinson DP and Klein SL. (2012) Pregnancy and pregnancy-associated hormones alter immune responses and disease pathogenesis. *Hormones and Behavior*, **62**, 263.

Sanghavi M and Rutherford JD. (2014) Cardiovascular physiology of pregnancy. *Circulation*, **130**, 1003.

Scriven MW, Jones DA, and McKnight L. (1995) Current concepts review. Musculoskeletal considerations in pregnancy. *Journal of Bone and Joint Surgery America*, **77**, 1465.

Sharma JB, Sharma S, Usha BR, *et al.* (2016) Cross-sectional study of serum parathyroid hormone level in high-risk pregnancies as compared to nonpregnant control. *Indian Journal of Endocrinology and Metabolism*, **20**, 92.

Sifakis S and Pharmakides G. (2000) Anemia in pregnancy. *Annals of the New York Academy of Science*, **900**, 125.

Silasi M, Cardenas I, Kwon JY, *et al.* (2015) Viral infections during pregnancy. *American Journal of Reproductive Immunology*, **73**, 199.

Soma-Pillay P, Nelson-Piercy C, Tolppanen H, *et al.* (2016) Physiological changes in pregnancy. *Cardiovascular Journal of Africa*, **27**, 89.

Stagnaro-Green A, Abalovich M, Alexander E, *et al.* (2011) Guidelines of the American Thyroid Association for the diagnosis and management of thyroid disease during pregnancy and postpartum. *Thyroid*, **21**, 1081.

Stjernholm YV, Nyberg A, Cardell M, *et al.* (2016) Circulating maternal cortisol levels during vaginal delivery and elective cesarean section. *Archives of Gynecology and Obstetrics*, **294**, 267.

Tenholder MF and South-Paul JE. (1989) Dyspnea in pregnancy. *Chest*, **96**, 381.

Thornburg KL, Jacobson SL, Giraud GD, *et al.* (2000) Hemodynamic changes in pregnancy. *Seminars in Perinatology*, **24**, 11.

Thornton P and Douglas J. (2010) Coagulation in pregnancy. *Best Practice and Research in Clinical Obstetrics and Gynaecology*, **24**, 339.

Tunzi M and Gray GR. (2007) Common skin conditions during pregnancy. *American Family Physician*, **75**, 211.

Uchikova EH and Ledjev II. (2005) Changes in haemostasis during normal pregnancy. *European Journal of Obstetrics, Gynecology and Reproductive Biology*, **119**, 185.

Vaidya B, Negro R, Poppe K, *et al.* (2011) Thyroid and pregnancy. *Journal of Thyroid Research*, **2011**, 1.

Zito PM and Bartling SJ. (2016) Dermatologic changes in pregnancy. *International Journal of Childbirth Education*, **31**, 38.

3

Implications of Physiologic Changes in the Dental Management of the Pregnant Patient

Christos A. Skouteris

The physiologic changes of gestation pose certain challenges in the dental and medical management of the pregnant patient. The challenges that will be discussed in this chapter are those that are of particular relevance to the dental practitioner.

Cardiovascular Changes: Management Considerations

As mentioned in the previous chapter, the physiologic increase in cardiac output is a compensatory mechanism to counteract the decreased oxygen capacity of maternal blood. Any event from any source that can cause a drop in cardiac output may result in maternal hypoxia and compromise the condition of the fetus.

The gravid uterus and its contents (fetus, amniotic fluid, and placenta) are of considerable volume and weight, particularly during the third trimester of pregnancy. If the patient is in the supine position in the dental chair or the operating table, there is a risk of compression of the inferior vena cava and descending aorta by the enlarged uterus. This can result in a decrease of venous return to the heart and a decrease in cardiac output by as much as 14% as well as decreased blood flow to the common iliac arteries. The initial response to the drop in venous return from the compression of the inferior vena cava is a

transient increase in heart rate and blood pressure. This response represents a compensatory baroreceptor reflex to maintain cardiac output.

The ensuing condition is known as *supine hypotensive syndrome* (SHS). The signs and symptoms of SHS are summarized in Box 3.1. Not all pregnant patients will develop symptoms of SHS in the supine position, but a substantial decrease in uteroplacental perfusion can still occur. Prevention and management of SHS are achieved by placing the patient in the dental chair in a semi-reclining position (approximately 30°), preferably with 5–15° of tilt to the left side, using a pillow or a wedge that produces a 10–12 cm lift of the right hip (Figure 3.1). If the symptoms persist or worsen, the patient should be placed in the full lateral decubitus position.

Respiratory Changes: Management Considerations

A pregnant woman has an impaired ability to tolerate episodes of apnea, pulmonary congestion, or excess nasopharyngeal secretions. Because of the effects of hyperventilation, a pregnant patient can present with a mild respiratory alkalosis (pH 7.40–7.46). There is also a postural effect that must be considered. When placed in the supine position, moderate hypoxia was observed in 25% of

Box 3.1 Supine hypotensive syndrome (SHS): signs and symptoms.
• Hypotension • Tachycardia • Pallor • Diaphoresis • Nausea • Dizziness • Syncope

Box 3.2 Respiratory changes: treatment considerations.
• Patient positioning as per prevention of SHS • Short duration appointments • Short breaks during dental treatment • Adequate suctioning of the oral cavity during dental treatment • Fingertip pulse oximeter SiO_2 monitoring • Supplemental O_2 (3 L/min)

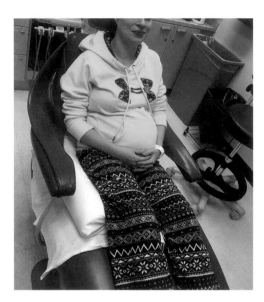

Figure 3.1 The patient is placed in a semi-reclining position with a 5–15° tilt to the left.

gravid women. Moreover, the supine position was also associated with an abnormal alveolar-arterial oxygen tension gradient that significantly improved when women shifted back to the sitting position.

Therefore, patient position must be adjusted for the pregnant patient so as to avoid hypoxia. Avoidance of long appointments, short breaks, and adequate suctioning of the oral cavity during dental treatment, basic noninvasive oxygen saturation (SiO_2) monitoring using a fingertip pulse oximeter, and supplemental oxygen via a nasal cannula are simple measures that can prevent hypoxia and improve patient comfort and compliance (Box 3.2).

Hematologic Changes: Management Considerations

The increased levels of clotting factors I, II, VII, VIII, IX, X, and XI and the decreased levels of factors XII and XIII result in pregnant women being in a hypercoagulable state. This produces a five-fold increase in the risk of thromboembolic events during pregnancy compared with nonpregnant women. Multiparous women are at even higher risk for thromboembolism. It has been shown that approximately 0.10% of pregnant patients have thrombus formation and up to 20% of these women develop pulmonary embolism, with a 12–15% mortality rate. The increased risk arises not only because of the maternal hypercoagulable state but also because of the compression of the vena cava by the uterus, with decreased venous return from the lower extremities. This results in venous stasis and predisposes patients to thrombus formation. Therefore, *the supine position should be avoided.*

Anticoagulant prophylaxis is recommended for pregnant patients with a history of thromboembolic disease (Box 3.3). For these patients, low molecular weight heparin is preferred because it does not cross the placenta (unlike Coumadin®), has a much more predictable dose response because of low protein binding (unlike unfractionated heparin), and has been demonstrated to be more effective than heparin for prophylaxis and less likely to

---

Box 3.3 Hematologic changes: treatment considerations.

- Patient positioning as per prevention of SHS
- Patients with a history of thromboembolism should be treated in a hospital environment

Principles of thromboprophylaxis in pregnancy

Low molecular weight heparin (LMWH)
- LMWHs are the agents of choice for antenatal and postnatal thromboprophylaxis
- It is only necessary to monitor the platelet count if the woman has had prior exposure to unfractionated heparin (UFH)
- Doses of LMWH should be reduced in women with renal impairment
- LMWH is safe when breastfeeding

Unfractionated heparin (UFH)
- In women at very high risk of thrombosis, UFH may be used peripartum in preference to LMWH where there is an increased risk of hemorrhage

- If UFH is used, the platelet count should be monitored every 2–3 days from days 4–14 or until heparin is stopped

Warfarin
- Warfarin use in pregnancy is restricted to the few situations where heparin is considered unsuitable, e.g., some women with mechanical heart valves
- Women receiving long-term anticoagulation with warfarin can be converted from LMWH to warfarin post partum when the risk of hemorrhage is reduced, usually 5–7 days after delivery
- Warfarin is safe when breastfeeding

Factor Xa inhibitors (e.g., rivaroxaban, apixaban)
- There is limited information about the use of newer pharmacological agents during pregnancy and their safety while breastfeeding

Source: Royal College of Obstetricians and Gynaecologists (2015).

---

cause major spontaneous bleeding. Treatment of an acute thromboembolic event will not be discussed as it is beyond the scope of this chapter.

Gastrointestinal Changes: Management Considerations

Nausea, vomiting, and pyrosis are important gastrointestinal manifestations during pregnancy that should be given special consideration (Box 3.4). For the pregnant patient with frequent or excessive vomiting, morning appointments should not be scheduled. Patients also should be advised to avoid foods that could initiate nausea/vomiting, especially fatty foods, prior to their appointment as they may cause gastric upset or delay gastric emptying. Frequent episodes of vomiting can result in dehydration and

---

Box 3.4 Gastrointestinal changes: treatment considerations.

- Patient positioning as per prevention of SHS
- Advise patient to avoid consuming fatty foods prior to appointment
- Advise patient to drink electrolyte-rich fluids
- For patients with nausea, vomiting, hyperemesis gravidarum, or gastric reflux during late pregnancy, the use of antacids or rinsing with a baking soda solution (1 teaspoon of baking soda dissolved in 1 cup of water) may help neutralize the associated acid
- Inquire about cannabis use if excessive vomiting is reported
- If marked extremity edema is noticed, refer patient to her OB-GYN for further evaluation

electrolyte imbalances. Patients with frequent vomiting should be encouraged to drink electrolyte-rich fluids, such as commercially available sports drinks.

Delay in gastric emptying caused by the decreased muscle tone of the gastrointestinal tract, gastric reflux, and regurgitation can lead to aspiration of gastric contents and, in some cases, death. It has been demonstrated that the acidity of the gastric aspirate is directly correlated with mortality. In this regard, prevention of aspiration of gastric contents during dental treatment should be the major focus of the practitioner. *The supine position should be avoided* because it puts the patient at risk of aspiration of gastric contents resulting from gastroesophageal reflux and regurgitation.

Liver changes of clinical significance include the serum concentration of liver proteins, particularly albumin, that can lead to peripheral edema caused by loss of oncotic pressure. Because of concomitant hemodynamic changes in blood pressure, extremity edema should be monitored carefully before and during treatment of the pregnant patient.

Genitourinary Changes: Management Considerations

Although frequent urination is often reported in pregnant women, true polyuria (>3 L/day) is rare. Given the increased frequency of urination normally seen in the pregnant patient, patients should be asked to void before starting treatment. Because of alterations in renal plasma flow and glomerular filtration rate, the doses of any medications that are cleared by renal excretion may need to be increased accordingly to account for their more rapid clearance (Box 3.5).

If procedures need to be performed under general anesthesia because of special circumstances, as discussed in later chapters, and placement of a urinary catheter is required, the patient needs to be evaluated for potential risk factors for asymptomatic bacteriuria: age of parity, sexual activity, presence of sickle cell trait, and low socioeconomic status.

Box 3.5 Genitourinary changes: treatment considerations.

- Ask patient to use the bathroom before starting treatment
- Adjust dose of medications cleared through the kidneys
- Weigh UTI risk before urinary catheter placement

Asymptomatic bacteriuria in the pregnant patient can progress to urinary tract infection (UTI) and eventually pyelonephritis, if untreated. Infections result from ascending colonization of the urinary tract, primarily by existing vaginal, perineal, and fecal flora.

Various maternal physiological and anatomic factors predispose to ascending infection, including urinary retention caused by the weight of the enlarging uterus and urinary stasis due to progesterone-induced ureteral smooth muscle relaxation. The loss of ureteral tone combined with increased urinary tract volume results in urinary stasis. Urinary stasis and the presence of vesicoureteral reflux predispose pregnant women to upper urinary tract infections and acute pyelonephritis. This is underscored by the distribution of cases of pyelonephritis during pregnancy: 2% during the first trimester, 52% during the second trimester, and 46% in the third trimester.

Glycosuria and an increase in levels of urinary amino acids (aminoaciduria) during pregnancy are additional factors that lead to UTI. The presence of aminoaciduria has been postulated to affect the adherence of *Escherichia coli* to the urothelium, thus increasing the risk of urinary tract infection.

Endocrine Changes: Management Considerations

Endocrine gestational physiologic changes involve release of systemic hormones, which alter cellular responses to insulin and the maternal metabolism, allowing for elevated glucose, lipid, and triglyceride levels in the blood, which are needed to better nourish the developing fetus. Elevated levels of progesterone, estrogen, cortisol, and chorionic somatomammotropin are all related to increased insulin resistance among a mother's cells. Thus, there is a significant risk for pregnant women to develop diabetes.

Gestational diabetes mellitus (GDM) is defined as any degree of glucose intolerance with onset or first recognition during pregnancy. A fasting plasma glucose level of 126 mg/dL (7.0 mmol/L) or a casual plasma glucose 200 mg/dL (11.1 mmol/L) meets the threshold for a diabetes diagnosis if confirmed on a subsequent day, and precludes the need for any glucose challenge. Approximately 7% of all pregnancies are complicated by GDM, resulting in more than 200 000 cases annually. Risk factors include marked obesity, personal history of GDM, glycosuria, or a strong family history of diabetes.

Control of gestational diabetes requires a combination of monitoring, dietary control, and human insulin supplements. Only 15–20% of GDM mothers require human insulin supplements, and most cases resolve following the end of the pregnancy. However, patients have an increased risk of developing type 2 diabetes over their lifetime, as well as a 30–60% likelihood of developing GDM during subsequent pregnancies.

There are numerous obstetric and perinatal concerns in patients with GDM, such as increased frequency of maternal hypertensive disorders, the need for cesarean delivery, and an increase in the risk of intrauterine fetal death during the last 4–8 weeks of gestation. Pregnant women with GDM are also at risk for numerous oral complications that require appropriate management (Box 3.6), such as periodontal disease, salivary gland dysfunction (xerostomia, salivary stones, sialadenitis), infection, neuropathy, and poor healing. Prevention and management of these conditions will be discussed in following chapters.

Box 3.6 Endocrine changes and gestational diabetes: treatment considerations.

- Encourage dental hygiene
- Prevention and treatment of periodontal disease
- Management of xerostomia
- Aggressive treatment of infections

Immunologic Changes: Management Considerations

Pregnancy is a unique immune condition that is modulated, but not suppressed. However, pregnant women are susceptible to infections. This is not only caused by a modulation of cell-mediated immune function that may result in a delayed immune response to infection, but also by other factors (e.g., GDM). Therefore, oral, maxillofacial, and neck infections (odontogenic or other) should be treated promptly and appropriately to avoid any adverse outcomes for the mother and fetus. Treatment of these infections will be discussed in Chapter 6.

Dermatologic Changes: Management Considerations

Physiologic skin changes and disorders in pregnancy that can manifest clinically in the oral cavity and face and their treatment are summarized in Boxes 3.7 and 3.8.

Vascular skin changes and vasomotor instability can cause *facial flushing* and *edema*. "*Greasy skin*" results from increased sebaceous gland activity. *Facial hirsutism* in pregnancy is usually due to an increase in secretion of androgens from the ovaries and placenta.

Melasma (chloasma or mask of pregnancy) may be the most cosmetically troublesome skin condition associated with pregnancy, occurring in up to 70% of pregnant women. The precise etiology of melasma is unknown, but in addition to the hormonal influence of

---

Box 3.7 Dermatologic changes and disorders in pregnancy: face and oral cavity.

- Facial flushing
- Pemphigoid gestationis
- "Greasy" skin
- Facial edema
- Facial hirsutism
- Melasma
- Impetigo herpetiformis

Box 3.8 Dermatologic changes and disorders in pregnancy: treatment considerations.

- Melasma – advise sunscreen use
- Pemphigoid gestationis – oral antihistamines and topical corticosteroids for mild cases; systemic oral corticosteroids for severe cases
- Impetigo herpetiformis – systemic corticosteroids; antibiotics for secondarily infected lesions
- Symptomatic geographic tongue (burning sensation): magic mouth wash or viscous xylocaine (gel)

---

pregnancy, exposure to ultraviolet radiation is a key factor in the pathogenesis. Melasma resolves post partum in most cases but it may not resolve fully and may recur with future pregnancies.

Pemphigoid gestationis (PG), also referred to as herpes gestationis, is an autoimmune subepidermal blistering disease associated with pregnancy. PG usually presents with pruritic erythematous papules and urticaria-like plaques with grouped tense vesicles. These lesions usually appear around the umbilicus and then spread to the remaining abdomen, shoulders, and arms. Oral mucosal involvement is rare and is observed in fewer than 20% of cases. In the oral cavity, PG presents with multiple painful erosions.

Impetigo herpetiformis has been considered as a variant of pustular psoriasis that occurs during pregnancy, but the current consensus is that it is a form of psoriasis. Classically, it arises in the third trimester with the onset of erythematous, annular to polycyclic plaques with peripheral, herpetiform pustules that may coalesce to form lakes of pus. The distribution favors intertriginous (apposing skin surfaces) and flexural sites. The oral cavity can become involved with the development of geographic tongue (focal depapillation with yellowish elevated margins and contiguous build-up of hyperkeratotic papillae). The dorsum and lateral tongue surfaces are most commonly affected. Geographic tongue is typically an incidental, benign occurrence, but the association with pustular psoriasis of pregnancy is well known.

Musculoskeletal Changes: Management Considerations

Changes in the musculoskeletal system during pregnancy, although adaptive and compensatory, can be the cause of considerable pain and discomfort. Painful muscular lower extremity cramps are common complaints of late pregnancy. Changes in calcium and phosphate metabolism as well as increases in both vascular dilation and venous stasis have been attributed as causes of lower extremity muscle cramps and edema. Lower back pain, pelvic discomfort, and generalized back pain can result from increased mobility of the sacroiliac, sacrococcygeal, and pubic joints, increased weight resulting in larger strain on the intervertebral disks, and from the increase in the size of the gravid uterus which leads to lordosis and muscular strain. Studies reveal that close to 49% of pregnant women experience some back pain during gestation.

When a pregnant patient is sited in the dental chair, in addition to placing her in the position that prevents aortocaval compression and SHS, every effort should be made (e.g., with the use of cushions) to provide enough comfort, especially when the patient experiences frequent episodes of back pain. Under such circumstances, treatment appointments should be kept as short as possible.

Psychologic and Behavioral Changes: Management Considerations

There are many positive as well as negative emotions experienced by women during pregnancy and lactation that also dictate certain behavioral patterns. The health provider has to be aware of these emotions and their distribution among the trimesters of pregnancy (see Chapter 2). Considerable patience is required on the part of the health professional and empathy and reassurance should be directed towards the pregnant patient, particularly when they express anxiety, anger, ambivalence, and negative feelings about the changes in the size and shape of their body. Anxiety in particular can be channeled by the patient into various behavioral attitudes, among which is fear of dental procedures, low pain threshold, irritability, and even impulsive aggressiveness.

The approach to the patient during treatment should be calm, with explanation of each step of treatment as it progresses and avoidance of actions unexpected by the patient. Disturbances, interruptions, and noises should be minimized. Ambient temperature should be maintained at a tolerable level. The aversion to smells that pregnant women develop particularly during the first trimester should be taken into consideration as it is common knowledge that the dental treatment room often has a unique smell to it. This may stimulate the patient in a negative manner.

> Caution: Any type of therapeutic intervention should be undertaken in consultation with the patient's OB-GYN, particularly when comorbidities exist and/or the proposed dental treatment is extensive or complicated.

Reference

Royal College of Obstetricians and Gynaecologists. (2015) *Reducing the Risk of Venous Thromboembolism during Pregnancy and the Puerperium*. Green-top Guideline No. 37a. Royal College of Obstetricians and Gynaecologists, London.

Further Reading

American College of Obstetricians and Gynecologists. (2013) Committee Opinion 569: Oral Health Care During Pregnancy and Throughout the Lifespan. *Obstetrics and Gynecology*, **122**, 417.
Berg G, Hammar M, and Moller-Nielsen J. (1988) Low back pain during pregnancy. *Obstetrics and Gynecology*, **71**, 71.
Cengiz SB. (2007) The dental patient: considerations for dental management and drug use. *Quintessence International*, **38**, 133.
Cheung KL and Lafayette RA. (2013) Renal physiology of pregnancy. *Advances in Chronic Kidney Disease*, **20**, 209.
Dahle LO, Berg G, Hammar M, *et al.* (1995) The effect of oral magnesium substitution on pregnancy-induced leg cramps. *American Journal of Obstetrics and Gynecology*, **173**, 175.
Dellinger TM and Livingston MH. (2006) Pregnancy: physiologic changes and considerations for dental patients. *Dental Clinics of North America*, **50**, 677.

Diokno AC, Compton A, and Seski J. (1986) Urologic evaluation of urinary tract infection in pregnancy. *Journal of Reproductive Medicine*, **31**, 23.

Flynn TR and Susarla SM. (2007) Oral and maxillofacial surgery for the pregnant patient. *Oral and Maxillofacial Surgery Clinics of North America*, **19**, 207.

Goldie MP. (2015) *Understanding Gestational Diabetes Mellitus*. Available online at: www dentistryiq.com/articles/2015/02/understanding-gestational-diabetes-mellitus-and-oral-health.html (accessed 16 October 2017).

Johnson EK. (2016) *Urinary Tract Infections in Pregnancy*. Available online at: https://emedicine.medscape.com/article/452604-overview (accessed 16 October 2017).

Khan I, Ansari MI, and Khan R. (2010) Oral surgery for the pregnant patient. *Heal Talk*, **3**, 31.

Koelsch S, Wiebigke C, Siebel WA, *et al.* (2009) Impulsive aggressiveness of pregnant women affects the development of the fetal heart. *International Journal of Psychophysiology*, **74**, 243.

Kurien S, Kattimani VS, Sriram R, *et al.* (2013) Management of pregnant patient in dentistry. *Journal of International Oral Health*, **5**, 88.

Lee RV. (2000) Symptoms produced by normal physiologic changes in pregnancy, in *Medical Care of the Pregnant Patient* (eds RV Lee, K Rosene-Montella, LA Barbour, *et al.*), ACP-ASIM, Philadelphia, pp. 52–67.

Liu JH. (2004) Endocrinology in pregnancy, in *Maternal-Fetal Medicine: Principles and Practice* (eds RK Greasy, R Resnik, JD Iams), WB Saunders, Philadelphia, pp. 121–134.

Mikhail MS and Anyaegbunam A. (1998) Lower urinary tract dysfunction in pregnancy: a review. *Obstetrics and Gynecology Survey*, **50**, 675.

Page EW and Page EP. (1953) Leg cramps in pregnancy. *Obstetrics and Gynecology*, **1**, 94.

Shetty L, Shete A, and Gupta AA. (2015) Pregnant oral and maxillofacial patient – Catch 22 situation. *Dentistry*, **5**, 9.

Shimanovich I, Skrobek C, Rose C, *et al.* (2002) Pemphigoid gestationis with predominant involvement of oral mucous membranes and IgA autoantibodies targeting the C-terminus of BP180. *Journal of the American Academy of Dermatology*, **47**, 780.

Shuresh L and Radfar L. (2004) Pregnancy and lactation. *Journal of Oral Surgery, Oral Medicine, Oral Pathology, Oral Radiology and Endodontology*, **97**, 672.

Thomas IL, Nicklin J, Pollok H, *et al.* (1989) Evaluation of a maternity cushion (Ozzlo pillow) for backache and insomnia in late pregnancy. *Australia and New Zealand Journal of Obstetrics and Gynaecology*, **29**, 133.

Torgerson RR, Marnach ML, Bruce AJ, *et al.* (2006) Oral and vulvar changes in pregnancy. *Clinics in Dermatology*, **24**, 122.

Tunzi M and Gray GR. (2007) Common skin conditions during pregnancy. *American Family Physician*, **75**, 211.

Turner M and Aziz SR. (2002) Management of the pregnant oral and maxillofacial surgery patient. *Journal of Oral and Maxillofacial Surgery*, **60**, 1479.

Varon F and Geist R. (2007) Diabetes mellitus. Available online at: https://maaom.memberclicks.net/index.php?option=com_content&view=article&id=87:diabetes-mellitus&catid=22:patient-condition-information&Itemid=120 (accessed 16 October 2017).

Young GL and Jewell D. (2002) Interventions for leg cramps in pregnancy. *Cochrane Database of Systematic Reviews*, **1**, CD000121.

4

General Principles for the Comprehensive Treatment of the Pregnant Patient

Christos A. Skouteris

Recording of Pregnancy Status before Treatment

Ensuring that pregnancy has been considered prior to any treatment decision should be an integral part of initial assessment of all female patients of child-bearing potential. The practice of checking and documenting current pregnancy status before surgical treatment has been shown to be inconsistent and with complete lack of data relative to pregnancy status assessment prior to dental treatment.

A simple, reliable means of detecting an early pregnancy before treatment is surprisingly difficult to find. Determining pregnancy based solely on history and physical examination alone can be challenging. Because accepted practice is to postpone elective procedures during pregnancy, identifying these patients before treatment is instituted is very important, especially in the early phase of gestation when it is often unrecognized by the patient and physician, and the risks to the fetus are the greatest. Pregnancy testing therefore appears to play a key role in ensuring that both the patient and healthcare provider have the opportunity to make a more informed decision with respect to treatment plans.

However, three major questions are raised relative to pretreatment pregnancy testing.

- How accurate is the test?
- How many early pregnancies can be identified?
- Is the practice of pretreatment pregnancy testing cost-effective?

Human chorionic gonadotropin exists in two forms: regular (hCG) and hyperglycosylated (hCG-H). In the first 4–5 weeks of gestation, hCG-H is the predominant form. Currently available point-of-care (POC) urine pregnancy tests detect hCG-H poorly. Despite advertising that they are 100% reliable on the first day of pregnancy, they may yield falsely negative results until week 5, when hCG predominates and reaches the Food and Drug Administration-approved detection threshold of 20 IU/L. A patient may be 4 weeks pregnant with a negative pregnancy test, undergo treatment, and then in week 5, when her test becomes positive, ask why an insensitive test was used. Quantitative laboratory serum tests detect both hCG and hCG-H with sensitivities of 1 IU/L. However, they are more expensive, more time consuming, less likely to yield false-negative results, and more likely to yield false-positive ones when the total serum hCG exceeds 5 IU/L, the threshold used to diagnose pregnancy.

In a prospective study by Manley *et al.* (1995), 2056 women of child-bearing age underwent preoperative pregnancy testing when presenting for nonobstetric, ambulatory surgery. The authors reported an incidence of 0.34% previously unrecognized early pregnancies, all of which resulted in cancellation or postponement of the procedure.

Dental Management of the Pregnant Patient, First Edition. Edited by Christos A. Skouteris.
© 2018 John Wiley & Sons, Inc. Published 2018 by John Wiley & Sons, Inc.

Azzam *et al.* (1996) reported the results of their institution's mandatory preoperative pregnancy testing in 412 adolescents, a patient group known to be reluctant to disclose sexual history or pregnancy status. No patient 14 years of age or younger tested positive but there was an incidence of 2.4% in patients 15 years of age or older. Older women may not be any more likely to know whether they are pregnant and therefore should also be tested. The overall incidence was calculated to be 1.2%. Similarly, Twersky and Singleton (1996) reported a positive pregnancy rate of 2.2% on preoperative testing. In a recent study, Hutzler *et al.* (2014) reviewed the results of 4723 day-of-surgery pregnancy tests performed at their ambulatory surgery center and acute orthopedics hospital over a 23-month period. All patients were scheduled for elective orthopedic surgery. There were seven positive results (0.15%) and one false-negative result (0.02%).

The cost–benefit ratio of preoperative pregnancy testing is a very difficult value to assess and quantify. A few studies have published costs of performing routine preoperative pregnancy testing. Manley *et al.* (1995) reported a cost of $2879 per pregnancy identified. In the study of Hutzler *et al.* (2014), costs were calculated using the charges incurred for a qualitative hCG pregnancy test. The cost per positive result was $1005.32. The authors concluded that routinely performing urine hCG pregnancy tests on the day of surgery is a cost-effective method of preventing elective orthopedic surgery on pregnant women. Of 4723 women tested, seven had a positive result and one had a false-negative result. The cost of $1005.32 for each positive test must be compared with an unknown – but very real – potential cost of an unfortunate maternal-fetal event associated with not testing. Should a miscarriage occur after elective treatment, or should the child have a congenital anomaly at birth, the health provider could be placed in an unfortunate situation that could have been avoided with simple pretreatment pregnancy testing.

The need for pregnancy testing before treatment was also clearly illustrated by Kahn *et al.* (2008), who reported that although they had to test 647 female patients to detect one true-positive result, with a cost of $3273 per true positive, this practice paid dividends because in the first year of testing, two women experienced miscarriages after cancellation of their surgery secondary to a positive urine test and a third patient with previous tubal ligation was found to have an ectopic pregnancy after a preoperative positive test result. Therefore, a dreaded medicolegal situation was avoided in the first two cases and a potentially devastating complication of rupture in the third case.

Recording of pregnancy status before treatment: take-home message.

All existing data appear to lead to the conclusion that pregnancy testing should be considered for all female patients of childbearing age when the patient seems be unsure about her last menstrual period, is uncertain about the possibility of pregnancy, or her reluctant response and general demeanor, particularly when asked about the possibility of pregnancy in the presence of others (e.g., parents), raises a strong suspicion that pregnancy could not be ruled out. Treatment has to be deferred and the patient should be referred to her gynecologist with a request for pregnancy testing, who also should be the one to discuss the results with the patient. If the POC is in a hospital, the OB-GYN service should be consulted.

Diagnostic Imaging Modalities in Pregnancy

Ionizing Radiation Imaging

Dental X-rays, Cone Beam Computed Tomography (CBCT) Scan

Concerns about the use of X-ray procedures during pregnancy stem from the risks associated with fetal exposure to ionizing radiation. With few exceptions, radiation exposure through radiography and computed tomography (CT) is at a dose much lower than the exposure associated with fetal harm. Confusion about the safety of ionizing radiation imaging for pregnant and lactating women and their infants often results in unnecessary avoidance of useful diagnostic tests or the unnecessary interruption of breastfeeding.

The risk to a fetus from ionizing radiation is dependent on the gestational age at the time of exposure and the dose of radiation. The most common fetal effects of ionizing radiation are listed in Box 4.1. If extremely high-dose exposure (in excess of 1 Gy) occurs during early embryogenesis, it most likely will be lethal to the embryo. However, these dose levels are not used in diagnostic imaging. Secondary maternal effects like tissue stiffness limiting head and neck movements, oral ulceration, and osteoradionecrosis may develop, compromising childcare by mothers. There is a risk of abortion and carcinogenesis in radiation-damaged tissues, raising the

---

Box 4.1 Ionizing radiation effects in pregnancy.

Fetus

- Growth restriction
- Microcephaly
- Microphthalmia
- Cataracts
- Intellectual disability
- Behavioral defects
- Teratogenesis*

Long-term effects

- Childhood malignancies
- Germ cell mutations
- Sterility

---

*Teratogenic effects are extremely unlikely in fetuses before the second week and after the 20th week of embryonic age. The fetus is not at risk of teratogenesis if the dose of irradiation does not exceed the threshold dose.

possibility of another primary tumor developing later in life.

Exposure to any radiographic imaging required for management of the pregnant patient in most situations should not place the fetus at increased risk. The pregnant patient cannot be denied the necessary radiographic investigations. The ADA endorses US Food and Drug Administration (FDA) selection criteria for dental X-ray exposures. It states that "Dental radiographs for pregnant patients may be prescribed according to the usual and customary selection criteria." The fundamental principle that should be maintained at all times is that the patient should be exposed to the lowest dose imaging modality possible, while still achieving the necessary diagnostic data (ALARA principle – As Low As Reasonably Achievable). A full-mouth series of dental radiographs results in minimal radiation exposure with E-speed film and a rectangular collimated beam. Bitewing and panoramic radiography generates about one-third the radiation exposure associated with a full-mouth series. If protective measures like the use of high-speed (E-speed, digital systems) films, rectangular collimated beams, lead apron, and thyroid collar are used, dental radiography is absolutely safe for pregnant patients.

The use of cone beam computed tomography (CBCT) scanners has become an ever-increasing part of dentistry. CBCT scans provide a useful modality for evaluating dental implant treatment planning, dentofacial anomalies, craniofacial pathology, and temporomandibular joint disorders. Therefore, CBCT scans may likely be considered during the course of treating pregnant patients. It must be noted that there are two major differences that distinguish CBCT scanners from helical or "medical-grade" CT scanners. The first is that CBCT machines use a low-energy fixed anode tube to generate the flow of electrons, and secondly, CBCT machines only rotate around the patient once as they capture data.

The net result is that the patient is exposed to approximately 20% of the ionizing radiation dose as that of a helical CT scan. This is approximately equivalent to the radiation exposure from a full-mouth series of conventional radiographs. Obviously, the use of CBCT scans should be exercised judiciously and certainly lead aprons and thyroid collars should be used at all times. If CBCT is deemed to be necessary, then the best decision is to limit the field of capture as much as possible to only the required anatomic structure in question.

Box 4.2 summarizes the radiation exposure from ionizing radiation imaging modalities in relation to safe fetal exposure levels, background radiation (cosmic), and other diagnostic ionizing radiation imaging modalities.

Medical-Grade Computed Tomography

Use of CT in pregnancy should not be withheld if clinically indicated, but a thorough discussion of risks and benefits should take place. In the evaluation for an acute process, the maternal benefit from early and accurate diagnosis may outweigh the theoretical fetal risks. Radiation exposure from CT procedures varies depending on the number and spacing of adjacent image sections. CT radiation exposure in certain situations (e.g., pelvimetry) can be as high as 50 mGy but can be reduced to approximately 2.5 mGy (including fetal gonad exposure) by using a low-exposure technique that is adequate for diagnosis. With typical use, the radiation exposure to the fetus from spiral CT is comparable with conventional CT.

The use of intravenous contrast media aids in CT diagnosis by providing enhancement of soft tissues and vascular structures. The contrast most commonly used for CT is iodinated medium; although this can cross the placenta and either enter the fetal circulation or pass directly into the amniotic fluid, *in vivo* animal studies have failed to show teratogenic effect from iodinated contrast media use in pregnancy. The iodine content has the potential to produce neonatal hypothyroidism after direct instillation of ionic contrast into the amniotic cavity during amniofetography. However, the intravascular use of nonionic contrast media has been

---

Box 4.2 Radiation exposure from dental, head and neck, and other imaging modalities.

Risk-free fetal radiation exposure level: <50 mGy
Background radiation fetal exposure: 1 mGy*
Imaging modality radiation exposure (mGy):

- Single PA view 0.005
- Full mouth series (18 images) 0.035**
- Full mouth series (18 images) 0.171***
- Bite wing (4 images) 0.005**
- Panoramic X-ray 0.01
- Cephalometric X-ray 0.003–0.006

- CBCT (dentoalveolar) 0.011–0.674[+]
- CBCT (maxillofacial) 0.030–1.073[++]

Note: Above values do not represent fetal exposure from dental radiographs

Other imaging modalities: fetal exposure (mGy):

- Chest X-ray 0.1
- CT head and neck 1.0–10
- Chest CT 0.01–0.66
- PET/CT (whole body) 10–50

*Total dose throughout pregnancy.
**PSP storage or F-speed film and rectangular collimation.
***PSP storage or F-speed film and round collimation.
[+]Small and medium field view.
[++]Large field of view.
CBCT, cone beam computed tomography; CT, computed tomography; PA, periapical; PET, positron emission tomography; PSP, photostimulable storage phosphors.
Source: ACOG (2016), ADA Science Institute (2016).

reported to have no effect on neonatal thyroid function. Although it is standard pediatric practice to screen all neonates for hypothyroidism, this test is particularly important in the neonates of women who have received iodinated contrast during pregnancy. The guidelines of the American College of Radiology on the administration of contrast medium to pregnant or potentially pregnant patients state that it is not possible to draw a definite conclusion on the risks of intravascular iodinated contrast use in human pregnancies and recommend that it should be administered only if absolutely necessary and after informed consent has been obtained.

Radiotracer Nuclear Medicine Imaging

Radiation-induced malformations have a threshold of 50–100 mSv. Most standard nuclear medicine procedures produce fetal radiation doses below 50 mSv. The National Council on Radiation Protection and Measurements and the American College of Obstetricians and Gynecologists agree that the potential health risks to a fetus are not increased from most standard medical tests with a radiation dose below 50 mSv (mGy). Potential health risks may increase in radiation doses that exceed 50 mSv (mGy), depending on the dose and the stage of pregnancy. For most but not all diagnostic imaging studies, fetal dose (and dose in general) can be decreased by a reduction in administered activity (e.g., half a typical administration), with a corresponding increase in imaging time (e.g., double) to preserve image quality. Several studies that assessed fetal radiation doses following technetium-99 m and 18 F-FDG positron emission tomography (PET) scans found fetal doses significantly below the threshold for adverse effects of radiation exposure to the fetus.

As a general rule, when used appropriately, the benefits of nuclear imaging procedures usually outweigh the minimal risks associated with small amounts of radiation, even in pregnant patients.

Nonionizing Radiation Imaging

Ultrasonography

There have been no documented reports of adverse fetal effects of diagnostic ultrasonography procedures, including duplex Doppler imaging. The Food and Drug Administration limits the spatial-peak temporal average intensity of ultrasound transducers to 720 mW/cm^2. Ultrasound machines are configured differently for different indications. Those configured for use in obstetrics do not produce the higher temperatures delivered by machines using nonobstetric transducers and settings. However, the potential for risk shows that ultrasonography should be employed prudently and only when its use is expected to answer a relevant clinical question or otherwise provide medical benefit to the patient. When used in this manner and with machines that are configured correctly, ultrasonography does not pose a risk to the fetus or the pregnancy.

Magnetic Resonance Imaging (MRI)

Studies of children who were exposed to MRI *in utero* at 1.5 tesla do not demonstrate exposure-related negative outcomes at 9 months of age and up to 9 years of age. There are no precautions or contraindications specific to the pregnant woman. Although there are theoretical concerns for the fetus, including teratogenesis, tissue heating, and acoustic damage, there exists no evidence of actual harm. Possible mechanisms for apparent deleterious effects include the heating effect of magnetic resonance gradient changes and direct nonthermal interaction of the electromagnetic field with biological structures. Tissue heating is greatest at the maternal body surface and approaches negligible levels near the body center. Thus, it is unlikely that thermal damage to the fetus is a serious risk. In considering available data and risk of teratogenicity, the American College of Radiology concludes that no special consideration is recommended for the first (versus any other) trimester in pregnancy. Finally, available studies in humans have documented no acoustic injuries to fetuses during prenatal MRI.

Unlike CT, MRI adequately images most soft tissue structures without the use of contrast. However, there are diagnostic situations in which contrast enhancement is of benefit. Two types of MRI contrast are available: gadolinium-based agents and superparamagnetic iron oxide particles.

Intravenous gadolinium is teratogenic in animal studies, albeit at high and repeated doses. Gadolinium crosses the placenta, where it is presumably excreted by the fetal kidneys into the amniotic fluid. In the era of gadolinium-induced nephrogenic systemic fibrosis, this raises theoretical concerns of toxicity related to disassociation and persistence of free gadolinium. The 2007 American College of Radiology guidance document for safe MRI practices recommends that intravenous gadolinium should be avoided during pregnancy and should be used only if absolutely essential; furthermore, the risks and benefits of gadolinium use must be discussed with the pregnant patient and referring clinician. Gadolinium is classified as a category C drug by the US Food and Drug Administration and can be used if considered critical (only to be administered "if the potential benefit justifies the potential risk to the fetus").

To date, there have been no animal or human fetal studies to evaluate the safety of superparamagnetic iron oxide contrast, and there is no information on its use during pregnancy or lactation. Therefore, if contrast is to be used, gadolinium is recommended.

The water solubility of gadolinium-based agents limits their excretion into breast milk. Less than 0.04% of an intravascular dose of gadolinium contrast is excreted into the breast milk within the first 24 hours. Of this amount, the infant will absorb less than 1% from his or her gastrointestinal tract. Although theoretically, any unchelated gadolinium excreted into breast milk could reach the infant, there have been no reports of harm. Therefore, breastfeeding should not be interrupted after gadolinium administration.

Diagnostic imaging modalities in pregnancy: take-home message

- According to the ADA/FDA selection criteria for dental X-ray exposures, dental radiographs for pregnant patients may be prescribed according to the usual and customary selection criteria.
- According to the American College of Obstetricians and Gynecologists' Committee on Obstetric Practice recommendations regarding diagnostic imaging procedures during pregnancy and lactation:
  - Ultrasonography and MRI are not associated with risk and are the imaging techniques of choice for the pregnant patient, but they should be used prudently and only when use is expected to answer a relevant clinical question or otherwise provide medical benefit to the patient
  - With few exceptions, radiation exposure through radiography, CT scan, or nuclear medicine imaging techniques is at a dose much lower than the exposure associated with fetal harm. If these techniques are necessary in addition to ultrasonography or MRI or are more readily available for the diagnosis in question, they should not be withheld from a pregnant patient.

Medications, Substance Abuse, and Their Implications in the Dental Management of the Pregnant Patient

Drug Use in Pregnancy

The major concern of drug administration during pregnancy is the potential for teratogenic adverse effects because most drugs cross the placenta by simple diffusion. Thus, the dental clinician must make a clear assessment of the risks and benefits prior to prescription of medications to pregnant patients. This determination can only be made if the weight of the maternal medical condition, the fetus's exposure risk, and the need for medical treatment are evaluated and balanced.

The first concern should be *to determine if a drug is teratogenic in nature*. The period of maximum teratogenic risk is organogenesis, which occurs from the end of the predifferentiation period, which lasts 2–4 weeks from the last menstrual period, until the end of the 10th week after the last menstrual period.

In an effort to determine the risks associated with the use of drugs in pregnancy, in 1979 the FDA introduced a classification of drugs based on the level of risk they pose to the fetus (Box 4.3).

Drugs in categories A and B are considered safe for use, whereas drugs in category C may be used only if the benefits outweigh the risks. Drugs in category D are avoided with certain exceptional circumstances, while drugs in category X are strictly avoided in pregnant women. However, the current FDA system of classification of the teratogenic potential of drugs is becoming outdated. As a result, in 2015 the FDA replaced the former pregnancy risk letter categories on prescription and biological drug labeling with new information to make them more meaningful to both patients and healthcare providers. The FDA received comments that the old five-letter system left patients and providers ill-informed and resulted in false assumptions about the actual meaning of the letters. Based on this classification drugs are either safe, used with caution, or unsafe for use during pregnancy or breastfeeding.

The new labeling is an evidence-based system entitled the Pregnancy and Lactation Labeling Final Rule (PLLR) that allows better patient-specific counseling and informed decision making for pregnant women seeking medication therapies. While the new labeling improves the old format, it still does not provide a definitive "yes" or "no" answer in most cases. Clinical interpretation is still required on a case-by-case basis. The PLLR came into effect on June 30, 2015 but the timeline for implementing this new information on drug labels (also known as the package insert) is variable. Medications approved prior to June 29, 2001 are not subject to the PLLR rule; however, the pregnancy letter category must be removed by June 29, 2018. Labeling for over-the-counter (OTC) medicines will not change; OTC drug products are not affected by the final rule.

The A, B, C, D, and X risk categories are now replaced with narrative sections to include:

- Pregnancy (includes labor and delivery)
- Lactation (includes nursing mothers)
- Females and Males of Reproductive Potential.

The Pregnancy section will provide information about dosing and potential risks to the developing fetus and registry information that collects and maintains data on how pregnant women are affected when they use the drug or biological product.

The Lactation section will replace the "Nursing Mothers" subsection of the old label. Information will include drugs that should not be used during breastfeeding, known human or animal data regarding active metabolites in milk, as well as clinical effects on the infant.

The Females and Males of Reproductive Potential section will provide relevant information on pregnancy testing or birth control before, during or after drug therapy, and a

---

Box 4.3 US FDA pregnancy risk categories for pharmacologic agents.

A	Human pregnancy studies are available and demonstrate no risk to the fetus.
B	Animal studies demonstrate no fetal risk but human studies are inadequate to determine risk.
C	Animal studies demonstrate fetal toxicity but human studies are inadequate. The benefit of use may exceed the risk.
D	Human studies demonstrate fetal toxicity. The benefit of use may exceed the risk.
X	Fetal abnormalities have been demonstrated in humans. The benefit does not exceed the risk.

medication's effect on fertility or pregnancy loss will be provided when available.

Regardless of how and when the PLLR will be implemented, it is still incumbent upon both the patient and healthcare provider to make an informed choice. The new labeling system aims at providing evidence-based information in an effort to disperse misconceptions among health providers and patients that all medications may be harmful to the unborn child. The risk here is that certain maternal medical conditions, if left untreated, may be more detrimental to the fetus. This may lead to progressive maternal disease status, teratogenesis, impaired fetal growth or development, premature birth, spontaneous miscarriage, or abortion.

When the decision has been made to treat the dental or medical condition of the pregnant patient, consideration should be given to the following.

- Selection of a medication must be balanced by the available therapeutic options.
- The degree of control required for a medical condition.
- The potential and degree of fetus exposure.
- The maternal and fetal risks of various medications.
- Dosages necessary for control and safety.
- Long-term effects of the medication on the fetus.
- Reviewing nonpharmacologic treatments.
- Becoming familiar with current pharmacologic standards of care.
- Considering older pharmaceutical treatments that have a longer safety record.
- Use scientific literature and study reviews.
- Confer with the patient's obstetrician, physicians, or pharmacists.
- Make use of reliable published reference sources, such as PLLR when it comes into effect.

The next concern should be the *degree of fetal exposure to a medication*. Not all drugs readily pass through the placental barrier. Drugs that bind to proteins or have a large molecule structure cannot cross the placental barrier. Drugs that could readily cross this barrier include lipid-binding drugs, acidic

medications, and those that depend on renal clearance. Physiologic changes in pregnancy can alter the pharmacokinetics of a drug. Increases in cardiac output, circulating blood volume, and vasodilation lead to a larger volume of distribution of a given medication, increased hepatic drug metabolism, and increased glomerular filtration and renal drug clearance rates. The unbound free drugs can cross the placenta and drugs that are usually cleared by the kidneys do so at a faster rate. This leads to lower serum drug concentrations and lower effectiveness unless the dosage is adjusted. The pharmacokinetics of many drugs in a dental office's armamentarium render them generally safe for both the pregnant patient and the fetus. However, if a dental professional has any doubts about either dental medication choices or risk factors for pregnant patients, consultation with the patient's obstetrician is required.

Local Anesthetics

In most instances, emergency, preventive, or restorative dental treatment during pregnancy requires the use of topical or injectable local anesthetics. Pregnancy may affect nerve sensitivity to local anesthetics. The time required for 50% depression of the action potential of A, B, and C vagal fibers from pregnant and nonpregnant animal models was determined after the application of bupivacaine. Onset time for conduction blockade in each type of nerve fiber was faster in fibers from pregnant as opposed to nonpregnant animals and the differences were shown to be highly significant. Preliminary findings suggest a slowing of nerve conduction velocity in humans with the progression of pregnancy. Therefore, the need to achieve profound local anesthesia is very important. Effective local anesthesia also prevents the release of high levels of endogenous catecholamines due to pain and stress during dental treatment. A study by Holtzman *et al.* (2009) showed that high catecholamine levels may be indicative of excess stressors and/or predisposition to elevated sympathetic activation that contributes to increased risk of spontaneous preterm delivery. Therefore, local anesthetic selection, judicious use, and proper technique are of paramount importance.

At present, and until the new FDA drug labeling rule (PLLR) is released, selection of local anesthetics and other medications (antimicrobials, analgesics, etc.) is based on the existing FDA classification of drugs in relation to the level of risk they pose to the fetus. Lidocaine and prilocaine are given a FDA category B and thus may be considered the safest local anesthetics to give to a pregnant patient. Of these two agents, lidocaine may be considered ideal because of its lower concentration (2%) compared to prilocaine (4%), resulting in less drug being administered per injection. Mepivacaine, articaine, and bupivacaine are FDA category C, making them a less favorable choice during pregnancy. Among topical preparations, lidocaine is the preferred choice since it is FDA category B as opposed to benzocaine which is FDA category C. For topical skin anesthesia, a Eutectic Mixture of Local Anesthetics (EMLA) (lidocaine 2.5% and prilocaine 2.5%) is an acceptable option (Box 4.4).

Local anesthetics freely cross the placental barrier, so the issue of fetal toxicity must be considered. The main concern in a pregnant patient is overdose with increased vascular volume and permeability. The majority of amide type agents are bound to alpha-1-acid glycoprotein. Pregnancy reduces alpha-1-acid glycoprotein levels, resulting in increases of free local anesthetic plasma concentration and thus the potential for toxic reactions, especially in bupivacaine. Maximum allowable dosage should be reduced proportionally. The maximum recommended doses of local anesthetic preparations for dental use are listed in Box 4.5.

Box 4.4 Local anesthetic selection in pregnancy: FDA classification.

Injectable		
Lidocaine	B	Safe
Prilocaine	B	Safe
Articaine	C	Caution
Bupivacaine	C	Caution
Mepivacaine	C	Caution
Topical		
Lidocaine	B	Safe
Lidocaine +prilocaine	B	Safe
Benzocaine	C	Caution*
Tetracaine	C	Caution*

*Can cause acquired methemoglobinemia in pregnant women.

Box 4.5 Maximum recommended doses of local anesthetic preparations for dental use.

Local anesthetic	Maximum dose	Maximum total dose	Maximum # of cartridges
2% Lidocaine + 1:100 000 epinephrine	4.4 mg/kg (7 mg/kg)*	300 mg (500 mg max)*	8 (13.8)*
4% Prilocaine +/− vasoconstrictor	6.0 mg/kg (8.0 mg/kg)*	400 mg (600 mg max)*	5.5 (8)*
4% Articaine + 1:100 000 epinephrine	7.0 mg/kg (7.0 mg/kg)*	500 mg	7
0.5% Bupivacaine + 1:200 000 epinephrine	1.3 mg/kg	90 mg	10
3% Mepivacaine	4.4 mg/kg (6.6 mg/kg)*	300 mg (400 mg max)*	5.5 (7.4)*

*The numbers in parentheses represent updated dosages as they appear in *Malamed's Medical Emergencies in the Dental Office*, 7th edn, Chapter 23 Drug overdose reactions, St Louis, Mosby, 2015, p. 353. The number of cartridges in parentheses was calculated based on those dosages.
Source: Adapted from Flynn and Susarla (2007).

Vasoconstrictors provide constriction of blood vessels by activating alpha-1-adrenergic receptors. Their combination with local anesthetics provides hemostasis in the operative field and a delay in anesthetic absorption. Delayed absorption of local anesthetics not only reduces the risk for systemic toxicity, but also prolongs the duration of anesthesia.

Although the use of vasoconstrictors with local anesthetics during pregnancy remains controversial, judicious use of a vasoconstrictor is permissible. Epinephrine is the most common agent used for this purpose. There has been reluctance to use epinephrine with local anesthesia in the gravid patient. Most of the practicing OB-GYN providers in Michigan do not recommend the use of epinephrine in local anesthesia. The concern is that accidental intravascular injection of epinephrine can cause uterine artery vasoconstriction and decreased uterine blood flow. In animal models, the decrease in uterine blood flow occurs transiently, but the magnitude and duration of this decrease are equal to the decrease in uterine blood flow caused by a single uterine contraction. However, clinically significant doses of adrenergic agents must be avoided to preserve placental perfusion and fetal viability. In this context, proper delivery of preferably amide local anesthetics with aspiration techniques so as to avoid inadvertent intravascular injection is considered safe in pregnancy, with the ideal agent being 2% lidocaine with 1:100000 epinephrine.

Antibiotics

Antibiotics account for nearly 80% of all prescription medications during pregnancy and approximately 20–25% of women will receive an antibiotic during pregnancy. Box 4.6 summarizes antibiotic selection based on FDA pregnancy risk ratings. This box includes a broader spectrum of antibiotics than those usually prescribed in dentistry, because certain conditions (e.g., odontogenic, maxillofacial, and head and neck deep space infections) might require the administration of a combination of different categories of antibiotics.

The use of antibiotics in pregnancy is affected by maternal physiologic changes which may lead to pharmacokinetic alterations that can affect both mother and fetus. These changes, that include increases in total body water, blood volume, plasma volume, renal blood flow, and glomerular filtration rate, contribute to increases in volume of distribution of various antibiotics as well as increased elimination of renally excreted antibiotics. Alterations in gastrointestinal motility may lead to changes in absorption, oral bioavailability, and delayed onset of action of certain antibiotics. There are known changes in hepatic enzymes during pregnancy that clinicians may use to adjust doses, but current data are controversial as to whether these lead to clinically significant changes in drug metabolism and subsequent serum concentrations. Finally, decreases in albumin and alterations in maternal plasma pH are expected to lead to decreased protein binding and increased concentrations of unbound drug.

As a result of the aforementioned changes in antibiotic pharmacokinetics during pregnancy, dosage adjustment (increased doses and/or frequency) is required. Antibiotics reach fetal circulation via placental transfer, three types of which have been identified. A few antibiotics cross the placenta rapidly and equilibrate in the maternal and cord plasma; this type of transfer is termed "complete" and includes ampicillin, methicillin, cefmenoxime, and cefotiam. Antibiotics for which concentrations are lower in the cord than maternal plasma are said to have "incomplete" transfer and these include azlocillin, dicloxacillin, piperacillin, sulbenicillin, cefoxitin, amikacin, gentamicin, kanamycin, streptomycin, fosfomycin, thiamphenicol, griseofulvin, and even those with a molecular weight greater than 1000 kilodaltons such as vancomycin and colistimethate. Ceftizoxime is the only antibiotic so far known whose concentrations are higher in the cord than maternal plasma. This is called "exceeding" transfer. Most antibiotics exhibit incomplete transfer.

Box 4.6 Antibiotic selection in pregnancy: FDA classification.

Penicillins			Aminoglycocides		
Penicillin (VK,G)	B	Safe	Amikacin	D	Caution
Amoxicillin	B	Safe	Gentamicin	D	Caution
Amoxicillin + clavulanic acid	B	Safe	Streptomycin	D	Unsafe
			Tobramycin	D	Caution
Cephalosporins			**Fluoroquinolones**		
All generations	B	Safe	Ciprofloxacin	C	Unsafe
			Norfloxacin	C	Unsafe
Carbapenems			Ofloxacin	C	Unsafe
Doripenem	B	Caution	Enoxacin	C	Unsafe
Ertapenem	B	Caution	**Miscellaneous antibiotics**		
Meropenem	B	Caution			
Imipenem-cilastatin	C	Caution	Metronidazole	B	Safe
			Clindamycin	B	Safe
Monobactams			**Antifungals**		
Aztreonam	B	Caution			
			Nystatin	C	Safe
Glycopeptides			Clotrimazole	B	Safe
Vancomycin	B	Safe	Griseofulvin	C	Caution
			Ketoconazole	C	Caution
Macrolides			Fluconazole	C	Caution
Erythromycin (base form)*	B	Safe	Amphotericin B	B	Safe
			Antivirals		
Azithromycin	B	Safe			
Clarithromycin	C	Caution	Acyclovir	B	Safe
			Valacyclovir	B	Safe
Tetracyclines			Famciclovir	B	Caution
Tetracycline	D	Unsafe	Penciclovir	B	Safe
Minocycline	D	Unsafe	Chlorhexidine gluconate	B	Safe
Doxycycline	D	Unsafe			

*The estolate form of erythromycin is contraindicated in pregnancy.
Source: www.drugs.com

Penicillins

All penicillins and their derivatives, as well as penicillin combinations with beta-lactamase inhibitors such as clavulanate or sulbactam, have a long track record of safety, with the parent compound penicillin and the amin-openicillins (ampicillin and amoxicillin) having the most robust safety data. Of more than 3500 fetuses included in the Collaborative Perinantal Project, there was no increase in congenital anomalies or other adverse effects after exposure to penicillin in the first trimester. Penicillin remains the antibiotic of choice in treating the gravid patient with an oral infection.

Cephalosporins

Cephalosporins have a long history of documented use in pregnancy. They remain a first-line option for many infections in pregnancy with general use reserved for patients intolerant (not allergic) to penicillin therapy.

Their plasma concentrations are decreased in pregnant patients because of increased renal elimination so dosage adjustment (increased doses and/or frequency) is required.

Carbapenems
Carbapenem therapy should be reserved for pregnant women with infections that are resistant to penicillin and cephalosporin therapy with limited alternatives.

Monobactams
Due to current lack of data, aztreonam use should be restricted to patients with severe penicillin allergy for whom beta-lactam therapy is contraindicated.

Glycopeptides
Vancomycin is considered to be safe for use in pregnancy in the case of serious gram-positive infections, particularly during the second and third trimesters. No abnormalities, including hearing loss or nephrotoxicity, were noted in the fetus after at least 1 week of vancomycin therapy during the second or third trimesters. Because there is limited information available about vancomycin use in the first trimester, caution is warranted during this period. When used orally, vancomycin has little systemic absorption, and is not believed to cause adverse effects during pregnancy.

Macrolides
The macrolide family of antibiotics includes erythromycin, azithromycin, and clarithromycin. Unlike most other antibiotics, the macrolides cross the placenta only minimally. From the macrolide group, erythromycin in its base form is the one most frequently used for oral infections in patients with allergies to penicillin. The estolate form of erythromycin is contraindicated in pregnancy because it is associated with maternal reversible hepatotoxicity (cholestatic hepatitis).

Tetracyclines
Tetracyclines cross the placenta and when used beyond the second trimester, they can bind to calcium in the developing fetus and cause permanent discoloration of bones and teeth. They are contraindicated past the fifth week of pregnancy. Despite earlier reports, tetracyclines do not cause enamel hypoplasia, and they do not inhibit fibula growth in the preterm infant. Tetracyclines should be avoided in pregnant patients.

Aminoglycocides
Gentamicin is the aminoglycoside most widely used during pregnancy. It rapidly crosses the placenta, with peak cord serum levels of approximately 40% of maternal levels in 1–2 hours. There have been no reported congenital anomalies resulting from gentamicin and no reports of neonatal ototoxicity or nephrotoxicity after *in utero* exposure. Case reports of irreversible bilateral congenital deafness with maternal use of streptomycin in the first trimester have been described in the literature. Despite toxicity reports, short courses of aminoglycosides may be used in pregnant women with careful monitoring if the likely benefit outweighs the potential risk. Due to the risks specifically associated with streptomycin use, this agent should be avoided.

Fluoroquinolones
There is a suggested association with fluoroquinolones and renal toxicity, cardiac defects, and central nervous system toxicity in the fetus. Animal data have demonstrated bone and cartilage damage in the fetus. However, in a recent literature review, Yefet *et al.* (2014) concluded that fluoroquinolones may not pose the same risks to humans as they do to animals because of weak study designs, small sample sizes, and confounding variables in the published human studies. The data are still not adequate to support their use in pregnancy and therefore their safety is not established.

Clindamycin
Clindamycin is a lincosamide antibiotic which crosses the placenta and shows no association with congenital defects when administered during the first trimester of pregnancy. Evidence is lacking for using oral clindamycin late in pregnancy.

Metronidazole

The use of metronidazole in pregnancy is controversial. The reduced form of the drug is teratogenic, but humans are not capable of reducing metronidazole and so should not be at risk. Multivariate analysis showed no relationship between metronidazole exposure at any time during pregnancy with preterm births, low birth weight, or congenital abnormalities. Although it has not been associated with adverse fetal effects, it is currently recommended for use in the second and third trimesters only.

Antifungals

Nystatin and clotrimazole have not been associated with congenital defects. However, recent data raise the possibility that nystatin is associated with a slightly increased risk of hypospadias in exposed fetuses. The use of topical agents for treatment of superficial fungal infections is safe and efficacious. Some data, however, raise concerns with the use of various systemic antifungal agents, including griseofulvin and ketoconazole, which may be associated with fetal malformations and should be avoided in pregnancy. Fluconazole is embryo-fetotoxic and teratogenic in rodents and rabbits. Total fluconazole dose >300 mg should be considered teratogenic and remains contraindicated throughout pregnancy. A single low dose (≤300 mg total dose) of fluconazole does not increase the risk of congenital disorders and may be considered in the absence of a topical alternative after the first trimester. Amphotericin B remains the drug of choice for the treatment of deep and life-threatening fungal infections in pregnancy.

Antivirals

The accumulated evidence for the safety of oral acyclovir and valacyclovir, established from pregnancy registries and as a result of the Danish cohort study (Pasternak and Hviid 2010), does not demonstrate an increase in the rate of major birth defects when compared with the general population or an unexposed group. Data on the safety of famciclovir's use

during pregnancy are quite limited, and although it might not be expected to increase the risk of major malformations, it should not be the first choice of medication for treatment of herpes simplex virus (HSV) during pregnancy. In addition, topical antiviral preparations of acyclovir and penciclovir resulted in no increased rate of major birth defects during pregnancy. Limitations of the safety data on antivirals include a high lost-to-follow-up rate in the registries and the lack of prospective controlled studies. However, these data are reassuring, allowing physicians to offer pregnant patients either acyclovir or valacyclovir for treatment of primary or recurrent HSV infection, which not only treats the mother's condition but also reduces the likelihood of transmission to the neonate, without unduly compromising fetal safety.

Analgesics

Medications used in therapeutic doses for acute and chronic dental pain appear to be relatively safe in pregnancy. To minimize fetal risk, drug interventions should be initiated at the lowest effective dose, especially in late pregnancy, and analgesics should be selected only after careful review of a woman's medical or medication history. Box 4.7 provides a list of the most frequently prescribed analgesics that are indicated or contraindicated during gestation on the basis of the FDA Pregnancy Risk (PR) ratings.

Box 4.7 Analgesics in pregnancy: FDA classification.		
Acetaminophen	B (C*)	Safe (Caution*)
Aspirin	C/D	Caution
Ibuprofen	C/D	Caution
Codeine	C	Caution
Hydrocodone	C	Caution
Oxycodone	B	Safe
Morphine	C	Safe

*Intravenous acetaminophen.
Source: www.drugs.com

Acetaminophen

Acetaminophen (paracetamol) is the most frequently prescribed analgesic in pregnancy. Most of the existing studies have not shown any association of acetaminophen with increased risk of congenital anomalies and thus, it is considered to be the safest analgesic for use throughout pregnancy. For this reason, oral acetaminophen has an FDA PR rating of B.

However, in an observational retrospective longitudinal cohort study that examined the association between acetaminophen use during pregnancy and childhood behavioral problems, Stergiakouli *et al.* (2016) reported that children whose mothers took acetaminophen during pregnancy were about 1.4 times more likely to have behavioral problems and 1.3 times more likely to be hyperactive. Although this study created quite a controversy because of its design, limitations, and ethical ramifications, the data seem to at least point to a correlation or link. Because of the ambiguity of published data on the potential risk of acetaminophen use in pregnancy, in a 2015 review of analgesic use during pregnancy, including acetaminophen, the FDA stated that "reliable conclusions" could not be drawn from all the studies it reviewed because of design limitations or other problems. Nonetheless, prolonged use of acetaminophen may have a very small risk associated with it.

Thus, taking acetaminophen as advised, 500–1000 mg every 4 hours to a maximum of 4 g per day, is considered safe in the pregnant patient. Intravenous acetaminophen has an FDA PR rating of C due to lack of animal and human studies.

Nonsteroidal Antiinflammatory Drugs (NSAIDs)

Aspirin and ibuprofen are the benchmarks of the NSAIDs. Aspirin irreversibly inhibits COX-1 and modifies the enzymatic activity of COX-2 while ibuprofen inhibits the two isoforms of cyclooxygenase, COX-1 and COX-2. Aspirin, in analgesic doses, has an FDA PR rating of C/D because of potential risks of miscarriage, fetal vascular disruption,

gastroschisis (a herniation of abdominal contents through a paramedian full-thickness abdominal fusion defect), dystocia and delayed parturition (childbirth), anemia, increased bleeding diathesis, and premature closure of the ductus arteriosus of the heart (if used during the third trimester). Bleeding tendencies in particular, specifically intracranial hemorrhage, were found only in infants whose mothers had ingested 5–10 g of aspirin 5 days before delivery. No bleeding tendencies occurred if the aspirin was taken at least 6 days before delivery. Low-dose (nonanalgesic) aspirin (60–100 mg daily) is sometimes recommended for pregnant women with recurrent pregnancy loss, clotting disorders, and preeclampsia.

The antiinflammatory and analgesic properties of ibuprofen, although advantageous for use in dentistry, have a less favorable application during pregnancy. Ibuprofen is given a category B ranking in the first and second trimesters but in the third trimester it is given category D and should be avoided, especially during late pregnancy. This is because it has been shown that the use of NSAIDs and of the newer COX-2 inhibitors late in pregnancy may prolong the length of parturition through ineffective contractions during labor. There are also concerns of increased bleeding during delivery and premature closure of the ductus arteriosus. These fears were largely derived from studies on patients taking large doses of aspirin and extrapolations from other NSAIDs.

Narcotic Analgesics (Opioids)

Codeine Few studies address the safety of codeine use during pregnancy despite its extensive use as an analgesic and antitussive in the general population. The frequency of codeine use during pregnancy has been shown to range between 1% and 3.5%. In the United States, about one in five women (21.6%) filled a prescription for opioids during pregnancy.

Though there has been some concern about the teratogenicity of opioids, the evidence of codeine teratogenicity in animal models is inconclusive. Few studies have addressed the safety of codeine use during human pregnancy. Epidemiological studies have shown a concerning association between maternal codeine intake during pregnancy and birth defects. A case–control study from the US National Birth Defect and Prevention Study (1997–2005) (Broussard *et al.* 2011) reported statistically significant associations between maternal codeine intake in the interval from 1 month before to 3 months after conception and a number of congenital anomalies including atrioventricular septal defects, hypoplastic left heart syndrome, left ventricular outflow tract obstruction defects, and hydrocephaly. The Collaborative Perinatal Project reported an increased risk of respiratory malformations associated with codeine, but not with other opioids (Slone *et al.* 1997). One case–control study of 504 children with neuroblastoma found an association with *in utero* exposure to codeine (Cook *et al.* 2004). Another study of 599 infants found that mothers who gave birth to infants with cleft palate or cleft lip with or without cleft palate used opioid analgesics (mainly codeine) much more frequently than the control group (Saxen 1975); the largest difference was seen for codeine use during the first trimester. In a third case–control study of 1370 infants, 12 infants with major congenital malformations had been exposed to codeine during the first trimester compared with seven in the control group (Bracken and Holford 1981).

Neonatal abstinence syndrome (NAS) has been described in two cases in which codeine was used by the mother over a period of several days close to term. Two other reports described an association between NAS and possible cerebral infarction after maternal intake of codeine close to term. Nezvalová-Henriksen *et al.* (2012) evaluated the pregnancy outcomes of 2666 women who used codeine during pregnancy. No effects of maternal codeine intake during pregnancy were observed on infant survival or congenital malformation rate. However, the association of codeine intake with acute Cesarean

delivery, atonic uterus, and postpartum hemorrhage may justify a certain level of caution when administering codeine toward the end of pregnancy. However, it is not clear whether differences in study design between the large cohort study and case–control studies might play a role in differences in the findings.

Despite inconsistent evidence, there are sufficient reasons to be concerned regarding the safety of codeine during pregnancy. Codeine and its combination with acetaminophen has an FDA PR rating of C.

Hydrocodone and Oxycodone Hydrocodone and oxycodone are commonly prescribed in combination with acetaminophen. Oxycodone is the safest as it has a category B ranking, indicating no evidence of harm to the fetus from animal studies and the absence of well-controlled human studies. However, in one study oxycodone showed an association with higher prevalence of preterm birth in exposed than unexposed neonates. In another study, neonates exposed to hydrocodone and oxycodone during pregnancy were more likely to be small for gestational age (SGA; defined as birth weights that fall into the lowest 10th percentile at each gestational age and can be useful at detecting exposures that restrict fetal growth on a population level). The Michigan Medicaid study reported 332 newborns exposed to hydrocodone, 281 exposed to oxycodone, and 7640 exposed to codeine, all in the first trimester. The rate of major birth defects was 4.6% for the oxycodone-exposed group, 4.9% for the codeine-exposed group (consistent with the general population risk), and 7.2% for the hydrocodone group, which could have been influenced by confounding factors (i.e., maternal disease severity and concurrent drug use).

Finally, a study which evaluated infant exposure in pregnancy to a group of opioids which included codeine, hydrocodone, oxycodone, and meperidine identified a risk of conoventricular septal defects, atrioventricular septal defects, hypoplastic left heart syndrome, spina bifida, and gastroschisis (Broussard *et al.* 2011).

Morphine Morphine appears to be safe when administered for analgesia for short periods of time, although chronic use has been shown to cause fetal growth retardation and neonatal withdrawal.

Note: The data on opioid analgesic exposure in pregnancy should be viewed within the context of the multiple methodological challenges that the study of opioid use in pregnancy presents. It can be difficult to differentiate whether the underlying maternal condition requiring opioid analgesic use or the medication itself is responsible for any observed increased risk. Future studies should consider the nature and severity of the underlying maternal condition and address the potential for confounding by indication. Due to small numbers, studies often consider opioid medications as a homogeneous group and by doing so, any effect for a specific opioid may be missed. Larger studies are needed, especially to allow for assessment of individual opioids, as it is unlikely that all drugs within the class of opioid medications have the same mechanism of action on the fetus. Furthermore, studies should focus on precise exposure measurements, dose, and duration information, as well as on accurate outcome assessment.

Corticosteroids and Decongestants (Box 4.8)

Corticosteroids are used for the topical or systemic treatment of oral diseases and in oral and maxillofacial surgery. The potential teratogenic effect of corticosteroids has been the main concern regarding their use in pregnancy. Prednisone and prednisolone have been used clinically in pregnant women, especially for treatment of severe asthma, without adverse effects on the fetus. Triamcinolone and beclomethasone are teratogenic in animals but have not been associated with fetal defects in humans. They are safe for topical application but systemic use can harm the mother and fetus and thus should be avoided during pregnancy.

Pregnancy-specific complications that arise include premature rupture of embryonic

Box 4.8 Corticosteroids and decongestants in pregnancy: FDA classification.

Glucocorticoids		
Betamethasone	C	
Dexamethasone	C	
Fludrocortisone	C	Unsafe during the first trimester of pregnancy
Hydrocortisone	C	
Methylprednisolone	C	
Prednisolone	C	
Prednisone	C	
Triamcinolone	C	
Decongestants (inhaled)		
Pseudoephedrine	B	Safe
Oxymetazoline	C	Safe

Source: www.drugs.com

membranes, reduced birth weight, increased risk of preeclampsia, hypertension, gestational diabetes mellitus, and lip and palate clefts. Weeks 1–4 and 5–8 after conception were associated with the highest increase in risk of cleft lip and palate. The evidence suggests there may be a small but significant association between systemic corticosteroid use and cleft lip and palate, but the absolute risk is small. The Collaborative Perinatal Project monitored 50 282 mother–child pairs, 34 of whom had first-trimester exposure to cortisone (Slone *et al.* 1997). No evidence of a relationship to congenital defects was observed.

In summary, corticosteroids should be used during pregnancy only if the potential benefit justifies the potential risk to the fetus. Their use during the first trimester should be avoided.

Administration of both inhaled and oral *decongestants* occurs during pregnancy. Decongestants are among the medications used in the management of odontogenic sinusitis and following closure of oroantral communications. Pseudoephedrine and phenylephrine are the most common oral

OTC decongestants, with 25% of pregnant women using pseudoephedrine as their oral decongestant of choice. However, oral decongestant use in the first trimester should be avoided due to their association with small increases in risk of gastroschisis, small intestinal atresia, and hemifacial microsomia. Inhaled decongestants such as oxymetazoline and phenylephrine are both category C and appear to be safe.

Some association seems to exist between oxymetazoline exposure during the second trimester and renal collecting system anomalies. These findings are somewhat consistent in terms of magnitude of effect and suggest that risks are even greater among women also exposed to the vasoconstrictive effects of cigarette smoking. There are, however, limitations to these studies, including the possibility of inaccurate recall of exposures and confounding by indication. In addition, the majority of decongestant use is in oral form and the question of whether intranasal formulations carry risk has not been adequately addressed.

Over-the-Counter Medications, Smoking, and Substance Abuse in Pregnancy

OTC Medications

Many pregnant women take OTC medications despite the absence of randomized controlled trials to guide their use during pregnancy. Most data come from case–control and cohort studies. Most OTC medications taken during pregnancy are for allergy, respiratory, gastrointestinal, or skin conditions, as well as for pain relief. All OTC medication use should be discussed with patients, and the effects of symptoms should be balanced with the risks and benefits of each medication.

Because of the expanding OTC market, formalized studies are warranted for patients to make a safe and informed decision about OTC medication use during pregnancy. This is particularly important because of the inadequate evidence base and inconsistent guidance provided by internet sites that list

medications reported to be safe for use in pregnancy. Women visiting these sites are being reassured that fetal exposure to these medications is safe even though a sufficient evidence base to determine the relative safety or risk does not exist. Half the websites that provide drug information are missing a critical message that should be paramount – pregnant women should consult a healthcare provider about any medication being considered for use during pregnancy. The wide availability of 'safe' medication lists warrants a consumer demand for reliable information on what OTC medications might or might not be appropriate for use in pregnancy. Box 4.9 provides a list of OTC medications, their FDA PR rating (when available) and safety in pregnancy. Medications that have previously been discussed, which are also available in OTC form, are not included in this list (i.e., analgesics).

Herbals and Dietary Supplements in Pregnancy

Herbs are considered natural products and patients may not perceive them as risky. The FDA, in conjunction with the Dietary Supplement Health and Education Act of 1994, has recently begun reviewing the efficacy and safety of herbs. Controlled scientific studies related to herbs are needed. Medical and dental providers need to become comfortable with routinely querying their patients about herbal and supplement usage above and beyond the use of vitamins. Health providers should also reference available scientific literature regarding the risks and benefits of natural products. Unfortunately, locating controlled scientific studies can be difficult due to the sparse literature on their safety during pregnancy. Available sources of information on the safety of herbals and dietary supplements in pregnancy ought to be viewed with skepticism because, unlike regulated medications, no mandatory system exists for reporting the harmful effects of dietary supplements. Some of the more widely used herbal and dietary supplements are listed in Box 4.10.

Box 4.9 OTC medications in pregnancy: FDA classification.

Antihistamines					
			Rabeprazole	B	Safe
Diphenhydramine	B	Safe	Lansoprazole	B	Safe
Brompheniramine	C	Safe	Aluminum hydroxide	N/A	Safe
Chlorpheniramine	C	Safe	Calcium carbonate	N/A	Safe
Pheniramine	C	Safe	Magnesium hydroxide	N/A	Safe
Cetirizine	B	Safe			
Loratadine	B	Safe	Magnesium hydroxide/carbonate	N/A	Safe
Fexofenadine	C	Caution			
Expectorant			**Antiflatulent**		
Guaifenesin	C	Unsafe (first trimester)	Simethicone	C	Safe
			Antidiarrheals		
Nonnarcotic antitussive			Bismuth subsalicylate	C	Unsafe (salicylate content)
Dextromethorphan	C	Safe			
Antacids			Loperamide	C	Limited human data
Cimetidine	B	Safe			
Famotidine	B	Limited human data	**Laxatives**		
Nizatidine	B	Limited human data	Mineral oil	C	Unsafe
			Castor oil	X	Unsafe
Ranitidine	B	Safe	Polyethylene glycol 3350	C	Safe
Omeprazole	C	Safe			
Esomeprazole	B	Safe			

The mild OTC forms of topical antifungal, antimicrobial, and steroid creams are safe in pregnancy.
Source: Servey and Chang (2014).

Smoking during Pregnancy: Tobacco and E-Cigarettes

The known health risks of cigarette smoking apply to both the population in general and to pregnant women.

In the maternal oral cavity, smoking can cause halitosis, tooth and tongue staining, altered sensation of taste and smell, delayed tissue healing, gingivitis, precancerous lesions (e.g., leukoplakia, erythroplakia, submucous fibrosis), and oral cancer (see Chapter 6). The deleterious effects of maternal smoking to the fetus have long been recognized through animal and human studies. Animal studies have proved that both nicotine and carbon monoxide cross the placenta and cause dose-dependent direct effects on developing fetuses. Other potential teratogens found in cigarette smoke include cyanide, thiocyanate, cadmium, and lead. These substances may be directly toxic to the fetus and may have vasoactive effects, or reduce oxygen levels, which damages the fetus.

The known consequences of smoking during pregnancy include low birth weight, risks of spontaneous abortion, preterm delivery, increased risk of sudden infant death syndrome (SIDS), and cleft lip and palate in infants who carry polymorphism in the transforming growth factor gene. These infants, when exposed prenatally to cigarette smoke, have twice the risk of developing combined cleft lip and palate and 4–7 times the risk for cleft palate alone. Long-term

Box 4.10 Herbals and dietary supplements in pregnancy: FDA classification.					
Black cohosh	N/A	Unsafe	Glucosamine	N/A	Safe
Blue cohosh	C	Unsafe	Goldenseal	N/A	Unsafe
Roman chamomile	N/A	Unsafe	Herbal teas	N/A	No data – Caution
Cranberry extract	N/A	No data – Caution	Juniper berry	N/A	Unsafe
			Mugwort	N/A	Unsafe
Chaste berry	N/A	Unsafe	Nutmeg	C	Unsafe
Echinacea	C	Safe	Pennyroyal oil	N/A	Unsafe
Ephedra products	N/A	Unsafe	Peppermint leaf	N/A	Safe
Feverfew	N/A	Unsafe	Passion flower	C	Unsafe
Garlic	C	Safe	Raspberry leaf	N/A	Safe
Ginger	C	Safe	Rue	N/A	Unsafe
Ginkgo biloba	C	Unsafe	St John's wort	C	No data – Caution
Ginseng	B	Unsafe	Valerian	B	No data – Caution

Source: American Pregnancy Association (2017), Dellinger and Livingston (2006).

effects in children who were exposed to maternal smoking during pregnancy have also been reported as increased risk for mental retardation, attention deficit/hyperactivity disorder (ADHD), increased prevalence of dental caries, and fluctuating dental asymmetry when there is a combination of maternal obesity and smoking. Fluctuating asymmetry is defined as the random deviation from perfect symmetry and is a widely used population-level index of developmental instability, developmental noise, and robustness. It reflects a population's state of adaptation and genomic coadaptation. The most widely used bilateral traits include skeletal, dental, and facial dimensions, dermatoglyphic patterns and ridge counts, and facial shape. Both environmental (diet, climate, toxins) and genetic (aneuploidy, heterozygosity, inbreeding) stressors have been linked to population-level variation in fluctuating asymmetry.

In light of the severity of maternal and fetal consequences of tobacco use during pregnancy, the need for smoking cessation is of paramount importance. Even women who used smokeless tobacco (Swedish snuff) had increased rates of stillbirth comparable to heavy smokers. Successful methods for tobacco cessation include patient motivation as well as behavioral and coping counseling and the availability of educational materials. If this is insufficient, bupropion (antidepressant and smoking cessation aid) has been used with success in nonpregnant patients. The FDA has given bupropion a B classification for pregnancy risk. Nicotine concentrates in patches enter fetal circulation after passing the placental barrier and cause vasoconstriction of both placental and uterine blood vessels. As a result, nicotine has an FDA PR category C rating and nicotine patches should only be used when their benefits clearly outweigh the risk of smoking or other cessation methods.

The recent introduction of e-cigarettes (ECIGs) has led to the misconception that they are safe for use during pregnancy as an aid to smoking cessation. The content of ECIGs is a liquid (E-liquid) which when heated up becomes an aerosol that the user inhales. The E-liquid contains nicotine, a variety of flavorings (such as cherry, cheesecake, cinnamon, and tobacco), ethylene glycol, propylene glycol, and glycerin. Although not studied during pregnancy, blood nicotine levels rise significantly with ECIGs and can reach levels similar to those achieved with traditional cigarette smoking. Studies have shown that of 10 products designated by the manufacturer as "free of nicotine," seven contained nicotine. It is the nicotine concentration of the product, and not the design of the nicotine vehicle, that mostly affects the baby's exposure. Ethylene glycol has known toxic properties and is not allowed in traditional tobacco products. Although the effects of propylene glycol on pregnancy have not been studied in humans, inhalation of aerosolized propylene glycol is known to produce throat irritation and dry cough. When heated up, the aerosol was found to contain formaldehyde, acetaldehyde (potential carcinogens), and acrolein which is formed from heated glycerin, can damage the lungs, and contribute to heart disease in smokers.

Not only have some brands of ECIG refill liquids been found to contain impurities at higher levels than permitted for pharmaceutical products, but also some metals, such as nickel, have been found to occur in concentrations 2–100 times those of cigarettes. Moreover, liquid chromatography-tandem mass spectrometry has revealed tobacco-specific nitrosamines present at 10 times the level published by the ECIG manufacturer for liquid refills. Potential adverse effects of these impurities on pregnancy are yet to be determined.

The efficacy of ECIGs to aid in smoking cessation has not been proven and ECIGs may be a deceptive smoking cessation tool. Although research has addressed the use of ECIGs in the general population, their use during pregnancy has not been studied. It is important for physicians and patients to understand that the contents of ECIGs are variable and not currently regulated by the FDA. Continued research is needed to inform patients about the potential risks and benefits of ECIG use, including during pregnancy.

Alcohol

The prevalence of alcohol consumption during pregnancy has been and remains difficult to quantify, given the reluctance of women to admit freely that they participated in behavior that society has recognized as risky and dangerous to the unborn child.

Health professionals should ask all their pregnant patients about alcohol use.

Ethyl alcohol is probably one of the most potent teratogens. The effects of pregnancy alcohol use are both wide-ranging and insidious. Any amount of drinking places a pregnant woman at risk. A safe threshold dose of alcohol during pregnancy has not been established, but current data suggest that binge drinking and chronic ingestion of large quantities of alcohol carry the highest risk for the fetus. Heavy drinking (>1 drink per day) has been identified as contributing a nearly five-fold increase in risk for low birth weight or birth length at or below the 10th percentile for gestational age, extreme preterm delivery (<32 weeks' gestation), miscarriage or spontaneous abortion. Women who ingest eight or more drinks daily throughout pregnancy have a 30–50% risk of delivering a child with all the features of fetal alcohol syndrome (FAS), which is characterized by several physical and cognitive birth defects. Alcohol consumption during pregnancy has also been found to increase the risk of fetal death. Binge drinking three or more times during pregnancy was associated with a 55% likelihood of fetal death compared to non-drinking pregnant women.

Fetal alcohol syndrome is the most well delineated of the consequences of alcohol use in pregnancy. The diagnosis is made by the presence of three features: characteristic pattern of facial abnormalities; growth defects, prenatally and/or after birth; and CNS abnormalities. Box 4.11 summarizes the clinical features of fetal alcohol syndrome (FAS, partial FAS, alcohol-related birth defects (ARBD), alcohol-related neurodevelopmental disorder (ARND)). Risk for these anomalies was more pronounced in heavy maternal alcohol consumption and among mothers who reported binge drinking (five or more drinks per occasion) during the first trimester.

The long-term dental implications for a child with FAS are mostly caused by the craniofacial disorders associated with the syndrome, but there is also a number of other

---

Box 4.11 Clinical manifestations of fetal alcohol syndrome.

Fetal Alcohol Syndrome

Cleft palate, multiple clefts
Microcephaly
Thin, broad or elongated upper lip
Microphthalmia
Hypoplastic vermillion
Short palpebral fissure
Absent or hypoplastic filtrum
Epicanthal folds
Flattened nasal bridge
Short nasal dorsum
Hypoplastic midface
Micrognathia (Pierre Robin sequence)

Partial FAS

Shows some of the FAS facial characteristics Partial FAS is associated with:
- prenatal or postnatal growth restriction
- one or more CNS neurodevelopmental abnormalities

ARBD

Ventricular septal affect
Atrial septal defect
D-transposition of great vessels
Hypoplastic aortic arch
Conotruncal heart defects
Bilateral renal agenesis/hypoplasia
Vertebral segmentation defects
Scoliosis
Hip defects
Ptosis
Strabismus
Optic nerve hypoplasia
Conductive hearing loss
Neurosensory hearing loss
Atopic dermatsis

Hard and soft neurological signs
(seizures, tremors, fine and gross motor difficulties)
Brain structure
Communication
Academic achievement
Cognition (IQ)
Memory
Executive functioning
Abstract reasoning
Attention deficient/hyperactivity
Adaptive behavior
Social skills
Social communication

ARND

One or more CNS feature of ARBD plus:
Marked impairment of complex task completion
Language deficits in expression and comprehension
Behavior disorders
Emotional liability
Subpar academic performance

---

problems that greatly affect oral health, function, and the quality of life of these children.

- Tooth agenesis
- Microdontia
- Delayed shedding of primary teeth
- Delayed eruption of permanent teeth
- Perioral and masticatory muscular weakness affecting mastication, speech, and swallowing

- Mouth breathing resulting in xerostomia, higher incidence of caries, and gingivitis
- Prolonged and excessive drooling
- Unusual taste preferences for salty or spicy foods at an inappropriate age
- Tongue thrust (orofacial myofunctional disorder (OMD))

Alcohol consumption also has detrimental effects on maternal oral health. There is an increased incidence of dental caries, tooth attrition and erosion, periodontal disease, and tooth loss. Alcoholics pay less attention to their general health and hygiene, which accounts for the increased incidence of dental caries, periodontal disease, and associated tooth loss. Other reasons for tooth loss in alcoholic women might be their risk-taking and aggressive behavior which increases the potential for accidental trauma and tooth loss. The probability of traumatic injury is further increased by psychomotor impairment that accompanies acute intoxication.

Alcoholics are also at higher risk of reporting sleep bruxism, resulting in attrition of teeth. Individuals who consume large quantities of alcohol have prevalent dental erosion. It has been shown that 49.4% of patients with alcohol dependency suffer from enamel and/or dentine erosions which arise not only from the acidic erosive potential of alcohol, but also from high relativity between alcohol, depression, GERD, and smoking. As is the case for the general population of individuals with alcohol addiction, the risk for the development of precancerous lesions as well as oral carcinoma is increased in pregnant women who are heavy drinkers. The risk of oral cancer in heavy drinkers and smokers may be as much as 100 times more than the risk of people who don't smoke or drink.

Illicit Drug Abuse

Maternal drug use and subsequent prenatal drug exposure have reached levels of critical concern. The 2010 National Survey on Drug Use and Health (NSDUH) conducted by the National Institute on Drug Abuse (NIDA) reported a substantial increase in the use of illicit substances among pregnant women. The rates of current illicit drug use were 16.2% among pregnant women aged 15–17, 7.4% among pregnant women aged 18–25, and 1.9% among pregnant women aged 26–44. However, current figures are still considered a low estimate, as maternal drug use is frequently underreported. Fear, guilt, shame, and embarrassment prevent many women from disclosing drug use during pregnancy. As a result, pregnant women may avoid or delay prenatal care, further jeopardizing their health and increasing the risks to the fetus. Therefore, it is incumbent upon the health professional to query the pregnant patient about the use of illicit drugs in a way that safeguards privacy and confidentiality of information.

Marijuana

Marijuana is the illicit drug most commonly used among pregnant women. Although some progress has been made to reduce illicit drug use in the United States, marijuana use continues to increase. According to the Substance Abuse and Mental Health Administration (SAMHSA), as many as 11% of pregnant women report recent cannabis use. The use of cannabis by pregnant women is expected to increase following the legalization of its use. In eight states, Nevada, Maine, Colorado, Washington, California, Massachusetts, Alaska, and Oregon, the sale and possession of marijuana are legal for both medical and recreational use; Washington DC has legalized personal use but not commercial sale. Twenty-three states and the District of Columbia have passed laws allowing some degree of medical use of marijuana, and 14 states have taken steps to decriminalize it to some degree. In addition to the known effects of euphoria, relaxed state, sleepiness, increased appetite, short-term memory loss, impaired judgment and verbal skills, perception distortion, and slowed coordination, one of the effects of marijuana that is seen only in pregnant women is the cannabinoid hyperemesis syndrome (see Chapter 2).

In terms of the effect on the fetus, although there is little consensus in the literature regarding the effects of prenatal exposure to cannabis on fetal development or physical defects, several studies suggest that cannabis use during pregnancy is associated with stillbirth, preterm labor, intrauterine growth restriction, low birth weight, neonatal intensive care unit admission and in some studies an increase in birth defects (obstructive genitourinary defects, polydactyly, syndactyly, and upper limb reduction deformities). However, recent studies have found no increased risk for birth defects.

Exhalation of marijuana smoke poses similar threats to infant health as second-hand tobacco smoke, which has been associated with increased rates of respiratory illnesses during childhood including asthma, bronchitis and pneumonia, and more frequent ear infections.

There is evidence that cannabis exposure during pregnancy has the potential to affect the maturation of dopaminergic target cells. Disturbances in dopamine function have been associated with an increased risk of neuropsychiatric disorders, such as depression, schizophrenia, and drug dependence. Other neurobehavioral function disorders among infants exposed to cannabis *in utero* may include:

- exaggerated and prolonged startle reflex
- increased hand-mouth behavior
- high-pitched cry
- poor habituation
- disturbances in infant sleep-wake cycles
- delayed acquisition of visual-perceptual tasks and language skills
- increased levels of aggression
- poor attention skills
- deficits in reading, spelling, and problem-solving skills
- poor performance in tasks requiring visual memory, analysis, and integration
- poorer school performance
- moderate cognitive deficits
- decreased IQ scores
- reduced cognitive function

- decreased academic ability in adolescence
- poorer reading and composition scores on the Welscher Individual Achievement Test
- delinquent behaviors with lower "executive function"
- impulsive or hyperactive behavior.

Cocaine

Cocaine abuse remains widespread and its use among women of child-bearing age is prevalent in the United States. Cocaine crosses the placenta and the maternal use of cocaine results in a rapid distribution of the drug to fetal tissues with several times higher concentrations in organs than in blood. Fetal cocaine exposure is not without consequence.

Cocaine causes vasoconstriction and hypertensive effects, which can result in a preeclampsia-like syndrome, myocardial infarction, cardiac dysrhythmias, stroke, migraines, seizures, and sudden death in the mother. Cocaine also causes premature rupture of membranes and increased contractility of the pregnant woman's uterus, which may lead to uterine rupture. Placental abruption is the most commonly reported complication of pregnancy in cocaine abusers and its incidence is four-fold that of nonusers.

The effects on the fetus from maternal cocaine use include preterm birth, low birth weight, small head circumference, intrauterine growth restriction, and increased neonatal mortality rates. Additionally, fetal dependency on narcotics has been associated with long-term maternal cocaine use. Neonatal symptoms may also include irritability, gastrointestinal problems, tremors, and even seizures. Congenital anomalies include heart and vision defects, hydrocephaly, cerebral infarcts, and neurologic defects.

As cocaine inhibits the reuptake of dopamine, serotonin, and norepinephrine, the majority of research into the effect of cocaine on human development has been on the effect on the nervous system – both the central and the autonomic nervous system. Cocaine has significant detrimental effects on cognitive and psychomotor development. Children with *in utero* cocaine exposure have been found to have attention deficit disorders during childhood and unknown effects toward their maturation.

Heroin, Methamphetamine, and Hallucinogens

Heroin crosses the placenta and enters fetal circulation. Use of heroin during pregnancy increases the incidence of premature birth, low birth weight, respiratory ailments, hypoglycemia, intracranial hemorrhage, and infant death as well as the transmission of HIV to the fetus from the mother who practices needle sharing.

Methamphetamine (MA) use and its effects on pregnancy and infant have been less well studied than those of opiates, alcohol, marijuana, and cocaine. Case reports and retrospective analyses have suggested that methamphetamine use may be associated with a possible increase of defects of the fetal central nervous system, cardiovascular system, and gastrointestinal system, as well as oral cleft and limb defects. However, case–control and prospective studies have not confirmed these findings. Currently, findings do not support an increase in birth defects with the use of methamphetamine in pregnancy, but methamphetamine use is consistently associated with SGA infants and neonatal as well as childhood neurodevelopmental abnormalities.

Methamphetamine has been shown to have deleterious effects on the dental and periodontal condition (meth mouth). In a study of 571 methamphetamine users, 96% had experienced dental caries, and 58% had untreated tooth decay. Only 23% retained all of their natural teeth. Another finding of this study was that, although national estimates from 2011 and 2012 indicated a dental caries prevalence among adults similar to that of the study group, the untreated dental caries in the MA group was twice as high (27% versus 58%). Furthermore, the tooth retention rate in the MA group was roughly one-half that of the US general population (23% versus 48%). Another disturbing finding was that nearly 60% of the sample were missing

one or more teeth and 3% were completely edentulous. While only 8.5% of adults in the general population have six or more missing teeth, the study showed that the percentage of MA users with six or more missing teeth was substantially higher (31%). Dental caries incidence was commensurate with amount of MA used. Meth users 30 years of age or older, and women or cigarette smokers were more likely to have dental caries and periodontal disease.

The potential cause of the extensive tooth decay seems to be a combination of drug-induced psychologic and physiologic changes resulting in dry mouth and long periods of poor oral hygiene. Methamphetamine itself is also acidic.

Phencyclidine (PCP) and D-lysergic acid diethylamide (LSD) are the most widely hallucinogens. Both PCP and LSD users can behave violently, which may cause harm to the fetus if the mother is hurt during a violent episode. Frequent PCP use during pregnancy can lead to low birth weight, poor muscle control, brain damage, and withdrawal syndrome. Withdrawal symptoms include lethargy alternating with tremors. LSD can lead to birth defects if used frequently during pregnancy.

Neonatal abstinence syndrome (NAS) is one of the primary negative effects of illicit drug use during pregnancy. NAS is a generalized disorder observed in infants experiencing opiate withdrawal. Heroin, as the most addictive illicit drug, is one of the main causes of NAS. Although other drugs including benzodiazepines, amphetamines, cocaine, barbiturates, and hallucinogens can produce NAS, studies indicate that its incidence is highest among opioid-exposed infants. Signs and symptoms of NAS include:

- yawning
- inconsolability
- sneezing
- inability to self-soothe
- sweating
- poor sleep
- nasal congestion
- respiratory problems

- mottling
- autonomic dysfunction
- fever
- gastrointestinal dysfunction
- increased lacrimation
- increased muscle tone
- tremors
- irritability
- high-pitched cry.

Neonatal abstinence syndrome affects not only infants exposed to illicit substances, but also infants exposed to the treatments for opioid addictions (methadone and buprenorphine). Given that methadone is the treatment of choice for opioid addiction during pregnancy, the need for alternative evidence-based interventions to ameliorate the negative outcomes associated with NAS exists. Buprenorphine has been found to be a safe and effective alternative to methadone for treating opioid dependence during pregnancy (Kraft *et al.* 2017; Ling *et al.* 2012). Buprenorphine was also found to be effective in reducing NAS in newborns born to opioid-dependent mothers.

Effects of Illicit Drug Abuse on Maternal Oral Health

Pregnant women with heavy substance use are at increased risk for poor oral health for a variety of reasons, including limited access to dental care, poor dietary and oral health habits, negative attitudes about oral health and healthcare, and direct physical illicit substance effect on oral health. There are several mechanisms by which drugs can directly affect oral health, including increased xerostomia due to hyposalivation, poor diet and self-care leading to higher rates of dental caries, enamel erosion, and periodontal disease. Depending on the main method of drug administration, abusers show several oral and facial manifestations. Box 4.12 summarizes the oral health effects of different categories of illicit drug use in pregnancy.

Note: Although there is ample evidence in the literature that substance abuse during pregnancy has serious implications for the

mother, fetus, infant, and later in childhood and adulthood, there are many confounding variables that affect the value of many of the studies on this issue. Among them are the reluctance of the mother to admit to substance abuse, the concomitant use of more than one illicit drug in addition to smoking and drinking, and the fact that it is not always clear whether the adverse effects of substance abuse are caused by the substance itself or by the underlying maternal medical and psychosomatic conditions.

Notwithstanding the need for more longitudinal studies that would provide evidence-based data on the effects of substance abuse in pregnancy, it remains essential that the health professional should always ask a pregnant patient about the use of illicit drugs, smoking, and alcohol consumption.

Procedural Sedation (Oral, N$_2$O, Intravenous)

Oral Sedation

Oral sedation is one of the ways to alleviate stress and anxiety associated with the anticipation of a dental or a medical procedure. Benzodiazepines (BDZ) are the most frequently used oral anxiolytics. This class of drugs has been assigned an FDA PR rating of C and D. Triazolam is absolutely contraindicated in pregnancy because it carries an FDA PR rating of X.

Studies have shown that benzodiazepines may increase the incidence of cleft palate, central nervous system dysfunction, and dysmorphism after *in utero* exposure. There are few data on behavioral teratogenesis, with a few reports suggesting developmental delay. The incidence of cleft palate is based on the fact that neurotransmitters regulate palatal shelf reorientation. Gamma-aminobutyric acid (GABA) inhibits reorientation. The theory is that benzodiazepines, diazepam specifically, may mimic GABA, thus causing incomplete palatal closure. However, the data from these studies are not reliable, due to a secondary drug exposure variable in the

---

Box 4.12 Effects of illicit drug abuse on maternal oral health.

Cannabis	Opioids and heroin
Xerostomia	Xerostomia
Periodontitis	Mucosal dysplasia
Smooth surface caries	Burning mouth
Leukedema	Periodontal disease
Pulpitis*	Taste impairment
Oral cancer	Necrotizing gingivitis
	Eating difficulties
Cocaine (snorting)	Dental caries
Nasal septum perforation	Mucosal infections
Changes in smell	Bruxism
Chronic sinusitis	Candidosis
Palatal perforation	**Hallucinogens (PCP, LSD, MDMA**)**
Cocaine (oral use)	Bruxism
Gingival recession	Oral ulcers
Xerostomia	Tooth wear
Tooth erosions	Dental caries
	Topical use
Crack cocaine smoking	Mucosal edema
Lip and oral mucosal erosions	Tooth erosion
	Mucosal necrosis
Methamphetamine	**Methadone**
Rampant caries (meth mouth)	
Tooth wear	Xerostomia
Xerostomia	Tooth erosion
Tooth sensitivity	Dental caries***
Bruxism	
Restricted mouth opening	

*Adverse effect on pulp vasculature.
**Methylenedioxymethamphetamine (Ecstasy).
***Attributed also to sugary methadone solutions. Sugar-free solutions are also available.

---

patient pool. Moreover, these studies suffer from a number of methodological limitations such as lack of careful report of BDZ patterns of use in pregnancy, possible influences of recall bias, lack of controlling for confounding factors, and lack of data concerning possible major malformations in aborted fetuses.

Although chlordiazepoxide and diazepam are considered to be among the safer benzodiazepines to use during pregnancy in comparison to other benzodiazepines, from a clinical standpoint, general advice should be that BDZs could be prescribed to pregnant women with severe anxiety after carefully evaluating a risk/benefit ratio case by case and in consultation with the patient's physician. In addition, the lowest dose for the shortest time may be prescribed in early pregnancy (first trimester) to avoid the potential (even low) risk of inducing a major malformation.

Nitrous Oxide (N₂O) Sedation

The use of nitrous oxide or N_2O during the treatment of pregnant patients remains controversial, given the absence of prospective, randomized, blinded trials of such exposure due to ethical concerns. Numerous animal studies have demonstrated a teratogenic effect of N_2O. However, it is difficult, if not impossible, to extrapolate the results from animal studies due to species differences. Retrospective epidemiologic studies have shown an association between N_2O exposure and reduced uterine blood flow, reduced fertility, lower birth weight, and a higher risk of spontaneous abortion. Anecdotal reports have indicated risks of cleft palate development associated with short-term use of nitrous oxide in combination with oxygen. In theory, the risk of cleft palate could be explained as the result of the N_2O anxiolytic effect being similar to that of benzodiazepines through GABA inhibition of palatal shelf reorientation.

Unlike other inhalation agents, N_2O inactivates methionine synthase, which leads to inhibition of the conversion of homocysteine and methyltetrahydrofolate into methionine and tetrahydrofolate. In particular, methionine is an essential amino acid, and tetrahydrofolate is important in the production of DNA. As a result, it is logical to cast doubts when it comes to using N_2O in pregnant patients. The effect has not proved to be clinically significant in humans, but it has been suggested that all patients undergoing anesthesia with N_2O receive prophylactic doses of folic acid, methionine, and vitamin B12.

Most providers agree that N_2O should be used only when local anesthetics are inadequate and after consultation with the patient's prenatal care provider. One important consideration for pregnant patients is to avoid hypoxia, and as such, N_2O should be used judiciously. If used for nonelective dental procedures, it is recommended that its concentration should not exceed a 50% mixture of N_2O to oxygen. N_2O has not been classified into any category by the FDA.

Note: The N_2O concentrations in dental procedure rooms should be kept at the recommended exposure limit (approximately 25 ppm or 45 mg per cubic meter) as per the recommendations of the National Institute for Occupational Safety and Health (NIOSH).

Intravenous Procedural Sedation

The management of nonelective dental, oral, and maxillofacial conditions may necessitate the use of intravenous procedural sedation. Procedural sedation and analgesia involve the use of short-acting analgesics and sedative medications to enable clinicians to perform procedures effectively while monitoring the patient closely for potential adverse effects (Table 4.1). Physiologic

Table 4.1 Risks of procedural sedation (specific to pregnancy).

Condition	Effect
Maternal hypoxemia (mild, for short periods)	Tolerated by the fetus
Maternal hypoxemia (severe)	Teratogenic, fetal death
Maternal hypercapnia and hypocapnia	Fetal respiratory acidosis
Myocardial depression	
Uterine artery vasoconstriction	
Reduced uterine blood flow	
Hyperoxia	No human evidence of adverse fetal effects of short-term 100% oxygen administration
Hypotension	Decreased uteroplacental circulation
Fetal ischemia	

changes and certain pregnancy-related conditions (discussed in Chapter 2) which should be given due consideration in procedural sedation include:

- increased maternal oxygen consumption
- decreased functional residual capacity
- maternal hyperventilation
- decreased maternal $PaCO_2$
- decreased systemic blood pressure
- supine hypotensive syndrome
- increased cardiac output
- decreased maternal hematocrit
- reflux esophagitis and heartburn
- delayed gastric emptying
- increased risk for gastric acid aspiration.

The drugs most commonly used in procedural anesthesia are fentanyl, midazolam, propofol, and ketamine.

Fentanyl Fentanyl has an FDA PR rating of C. It readily crosses the placenta, and evidence shows that it is rapidly metabolized and redistributed in the fetus. There are no human data regarding the use of fentanyl in early pregnancy. Animal studies have failed to reveal evidence of teratogenicity but some reproductive toxicity has been reported.

Midazolam Midazolam is a benzodiazepine with an FDA PR rating of C. The potential effects of benzodiazepines on the fetus have been discussed under "Oral Sedation."

Propofol Propofol is the anesthetic of choice for short-duration surgical procedures because of its short action and rapid clearance from the circulation. Propofol has an FDA PR rating of B. Maternal hypotension is a common adverse effect of propofol, but one study showed that it has a dilating effect on fetal placental blood vessels, and therefore maintains appropriate umbilical blood flow. There is no animal or human evidence for teratogenicity of propofol; however, there are concerns about a transient depression of neonatal neurobehavioral function when propofol is used close to delivery, especially in high doses (9 mg/kg).

Ketamine Ketamine has an FDA PR rating of N (not classified). No human data regarding the teratogenicity of ketamine exist. Some studies demonstrated dose-dependent uterine contractions in early and late pregnancy, but others did not. These effects were more prominent in early pregnancy and with a maternal dose of 2 mg/kg or more. Ketamine is known to increase maternal blood pressure and heart rate by up to 30–40%, and it is therefore not recommended for use in women with preexisting hypertension. Neonatal depression of neurobehavioral function is also a concern when ketamine is given close to delivery. The limited available human data suggest that ketamine may be used in low doses throughout pregnancy, but other agents may be preferable.

Note: It is very important that the level of sedation should be closely monitored and controlled during the procedure. If the level of deep sedation has been reached, assistance may be needed to ensure the airway is protected and adequate ventilation maintained. If deep sedation is allowed to progress to the level of general anesthesia, intubation may be necessary. There is an increased risk of difficult intubation in pregnant women because of physiologic changes in the maternal airway. Loss of airway control is the most common cause of anesthesia-related maternal mortality.

General Anesthesia

Nonobstetric surgery can be required during any stage of pregnancy, depending on the urgency of the indication. The most common indications are acute odontogenic infections, abdominal infections (acute appendicitis incidence 1:2000 pregnancies and cholecystitis 6:1000 pregnancies), maternal trauma, and surgery for maternal aggressive benign and malignant tumors. When caring for pregnant women undergoing nonobstetric surgery, safe anesthesia must be provided for both the mother and the fetus.

Thorough understanding of the physiologic and pharmacologic adaptations of pregnancy is required to insure maternal safety. Fetal safety requires avoidance of potentially dangerous drugs at critical times during fetal development, assurance of continuation of adequate uteroplacental perfusion, and avoidance and/or treatment of preterm labor and delivery.

Airway changes include swelling and friability of oropharyngeal mucosa that contributes to increased incidence of epistaxis, reduced size of the glottic opening, and difficult intubation. Studies have shown that Mallampati classification (III and IV) is more predictive of difficult intubation in pregnancy than in nonpregnant women. The higher incidence of failed intubation during anesthesia induction in pregnant women has been debated in the literature. Whether or not failed intubation is becoming more frequent, the loss of airway control is the most common cause of anesthesia-related maternal mortality. Steps to decrease the risk of maternal airway loss during anesthesia include better clinical training with simulation, well-rehearsed airway emergency algorithms with readily available advanced airway devices, and experienced anesthesia personnel.

Pregnant patients have an increased risk for aspiration. Physical changes during pregnancy include increased size of the uterus, which causes a mechanical superior displacement of the stomach and increases intragastric pressure. These patients are also prone to increased gastric reflux, delayed gastric motility, and reduced competency of the gastroesophageal sphincter. The decreased lower esophageal sphincter tone may be due to direct hormonal effects of progesterone.

The use of general anesthesia in the pregnant patient, regardless of the agent used, has to address three very important issues in relation to the fetus: avoidance of teratogenic agents, nonreassuring fetal status (previously known as "fetal asphyxia"), and prevention of premature labor.

Avoidance of Teratogenic Agents

Despite years of animal studies and observational studies in humans, no anesthetic drug has been shown to be clearly dangerous to the human fetus and there is no optimal anesthetic technique. The largest retrospective study of exposure to surgery and anesthesia in pregnancy was conducted by Mazze and Kallen (1989) in which they evaluated data from three Swedish healthcare registries for the years 1973–1981. Of 720 000 pregnant women, 5405 (0.75%) had nonobstetric surgery, including 2252 who had procedures during the first trimester. There was no difference between surgical and control patients with regard to the incidence of stillbirth or the overall incidence of congenital anomalies. However, there was an increased incidence of low birth weight (1500 g) as a result of prematurity and intrauterine growth restriction in the surgical group and an increased rate of neural tube defects with exposure in the first trimester.

A metaanalysis evaluated 54 of 4052 publications that met the inclusion criteria, which included 12 452 women having surgery during pregnancy (Cohen-Kerem *et al.* 2005). The authors found that maternal mortality was less than 1/10 000, nonobstetric surgery did not increase the risk of major birth defects, and surgery and general anesthesia were not major risk factors for spontaneous abortion; however, acute appendicitis with peritonitis posed a risk for fetal loss. Table 4.2 lists the general anesthetic agents most widely used for induction, inhalation, and neuromuscular blockade with their corresponding FDA PR rating.

Nonreassuring Fetal Status

Nonreassuring fetal status results from acute oxygen deprivation. When maternal PaO_2 and $PaCO_2$, uterine vascular resistance, and blood pressure are maintained within normal limits, fetal oxygenation is assured. Fetal hypoxia can develop acutely in pregnant women during general anesthesia. This can

Table 4.2 General anesthesia in pregnancy: FDA classification.

General anesthetic agents[*]		Teratogenicity–Adverse effects	
(*Induction, inhalation, neuromuscular blockers, reversals*)		*Animals*	*Humans*[**]
Propofol	B	No	No
Etomidate	C	Yes	No
Isoflurane	C	Yes	No
Desflurane	B	No	No
Sevoflurane	B	No	No
Atracurium	C	Yes	No
Pancuronium	C	N/A	No
Vecuronium	C	N/A	No
Succinylcholine***	C	N/A	No
Sugammedex****	N	No	No

*Most widely used.
**No adequate/well-controlled human studies available. No teratogenicity or adverse effects observed.
***Use with caution in pregnant women with abnormally low pseudocholinesterase concentrations.
****Reverses rocuronium and vecuronium. N: FDA PR not assigned.
N/A, no animal studies available.
Note: The general recommendation is that each one of the listed general anesthetic agents should be used during pregnancy if there is no other alternative and only if the potential benefit justifies the potential risks to the fetus.
Source: www.drugs.com

be managed by oxygen administration. High levels of oxygen for a short period of time do not seem to cause any adverse effects to the fetus. The oxygen dissociation curve is left-shifted in the fetus (which encourages uptake of oxygen from maternal supplies), and the average Hgb in the fetus is 17 g/dL, so while fetal pO_2 is only ~30 mmHg, oxygen content is almost identical to that of its mother. A healthy fetus can safely tolerate a 50% reduction in oxygen delivery. Exchange of CO_2 depends on concentration gradients and uterine blood flow.

Placental vasculature normally exists in a vasodilated state (although not maximally so, as is classically taught), probably secondary to nitric oxide release. Many studies of uterine blood flow rely on the S/D ratio, which is the ratio of maximal velocity during systole divided by the minimal velocity during diastole – an elevated S/D ratio is associated with poor placental perfusion. Maternal hypocapnia (usually the result of hyperventilation and increased thoracic pressure) can cause nonreassuring fetal status, fetal hypoxia, and acidosis secondary to vasoconstriction, decreased venous return, and left shift of the maternal oxygen dissociation curve (CO_2 leads to unloading of O_2, hypocapnia leads to retention of O_2).

Maternal hypotension is probably of the greatest concern intraoperatively. Deep levels of inhalation agents will cause rapid maternal hypotension, which can result in fetal hypoxia. Therefore, lighter levels of general anesthesia agents should be used to attenuate surgical stress but not sufficient to decrease maternal blood pressure. If maternal hypotension does occur, treatment should be administered immediately. Treatment consists of intravenous fluid administration, repositioning the patient to a lateral position, decreasing the anesthetic concentration, and use of a vaso-constrictor. For decades, ephedrine was the drug of choice for the treatment of maternal hypotension based on classic studies in sheep that suggested deleterious effects of pure alpha-adrenergic agonists such as phenylephrine on uteroplacental blood flow. However, contrary to past recommendations, both ephedrine and phenylephrine are considered safe and effective pressors for control of maternal arterial pressure during pregnancy. Moreover, clinical trials in the last two decades have demonstrated that phenylephrine and other alpha-agonists (e.g. metaraminol) are safe and generally more effective than ephedrine alone to prevent maternal hypotension and its sequelae (e.g., nausea and vomiting). Furthermore, ephedrine use is associated with lower neonatal pH and a higher incidence of neonatal acidosis than the use of phenylephrine or other pure alpha-agonists.

Prevention of Premature Labour

A number of studies have reported on the potential association between general anesthesia and an increased risk of premature delivery. One study showed an approximate premature delivery rate of 9% with a 7.5% perinatal mortality. The norm for premature delivery in this study was 2.2%. Studies like this and others that compare general anesthetics and premature delivery have an inherent problem: it is very difficult to determine whether the incidence of premature delivery is the result of the general anesthetic agents or the effect of surgical stress on the patient. It seems more likely that the surgical stress is causing the premature delivery and not the general anesthetic agents.

Fetal Monitoring

The American College of Obstetricians and Gynecologists' Committee on Obstetric Practice issued the following recommendations relative to nonobstetric surgery during pregnancy.

- Surgery should be done at an institution with neonatal and pediatric services.
- An obstetric care provider with cesarean delivery privileges should be readily available.
- A qualified individual should be readily available to interpret the fetal heart rate patterns.

General guidelines for fetal monitoring include the following.

- If the fetus is considered previable (not sufficiently developed to survive outside the uterus), it is generally sufficient to ascertain the fetal heart rate by Doppler before and after the procedure.
- At a minimum, if the fetus is considered to be viable, simultaneous electronic fetal heart rate and contraction monitoring should be performed before and after the procedure to assess fetal well-being and the absence of contractions.

Intraoperative electronic fetal monitoring may be appropriate when all of the following apply.

- The fetus is viable.
- It is physically possible to perform intraoperative electronic fetal monitoring.
- A healthcare provider with obstetric surgery privileges is available and willing to intervene during the surgical procedure for fetal indications.
- When possible, the woman has given informed consent to emergency cesarean delivery.
- The nature of the planned surgery will allow the safe interruption or alteration of the procedure to provide access to perform emergency delivery.

In selected circumstances, intraoperative fetal monitoring may be considered for previable fetuses to facilitate positioning or oxygenation interventions.

The decision to use fetal monitoring should be individualized and, if used, should be based on gestational age, type of surgery, and facilities available. Ultimately, each case warrants a team approach (anesthesia and obstetric care providers, surgeons, pediatricians, and nurses) for optimal safety of the woman and the fetus.

Note: In the setting of general anesthesia, loss of fetal heart rate variability is not always an indicator of fetal distress, but may simply be an indication of expected anesthetic effects on the fetal autonomic nervous system. Slowing of the fetal heart rate in the operative setting is more concerning for fetal hypoxemia and acidosis, but could also be related to a decrease in temperature, maternal respiratory acidosis, or the administration of drugs, anesthetic agents, or both, which tend to slow the heart rate.

References

ADA Science Institute, Center for Scientific Information (2016) *X-rays: Radiation Exposure in Dentistry*. Available online at: www.ada.org/en/member-center/oral-health-topics/x-rays (accessed 18 October 2017).

American College of Obstetricians and Gynecologists (2016) Committee Opinion No. 656. Guidelines for Diagnostic Imaging During Pregnancy and Lactation. *Obstetrics and Gynecology*, **127**, e75.

American Pregnancy Association (2015) *Using Illegal Drugs During Pregnancy*. Available online at http://americanpregnancy.org/pregnancy-health/illegal-drugs-during-pregnancy/ (accessed 18 October 2017).

American Pregnancy Association (2017) *Herbs and Pregnancy*. Available online at: http://americanpregnancy.org/pregnancy-health/herbs-and-pregnancy/ (accessed 18 October 2017).

Azzam FJ, Padda GS, DeBoard JW, *et al.* (1996) Preoperative pregnancy testing in adolescents. *Anesthesia and Analgesia*, **82**, 4.

Bracken M and Holford T. (1981) Exposure to prescribed drugs in pregnancy and association with congenital malformation. *Obstetrics and Gynecology*, **58**, 336.

Broussard CS, Rasmussen SA, Reefhuis J, *et al.* and National Birth Defects Prevention Study. (2011) Maternal treatment with opioid analgesics and risk for birth defects. *American Journal of Obstetrics and Gynecology*, **204**, 314.

Cohen-Kerem R, Railton C, Oren D, *et al.* (2005) Pregnancy outcome following non-obstetric surgical intervention. *American Journal of Surgery*, **190**, 467.

Cook M, Olshan A, Guess H, *et al.* (2004) Maternal medication use and neuroblastoma in offspring. *American Journal of Epidemiology*, **159**, 721.

Dellinger TM and Livingston MH. (2006) Pregnancy: physiologic changes and considerations for dental patients. *Dental Clinics of North America*, **50**, 677.

Flynn TR and Susarla SM. (2007) Oral and maxillofacial surgery for the pregnant patient. *Oral and Maxillofacial Surgery Clinics of North America*, **19**, 207.

Holtzman C, Senagore P, Tian Y, *et al.* (2009) Maternal catecholamine levels in midpregnancy and risk of preterm delivery. *American Journal of Epidemiology*, **170**, 1014.

Hutzler L, Kraemer K, Palmer N, *et al.* (2014) Cost benefit analysis of same day pregnancy tests in elective orthopaedic surgery. *Bulletin of the NYU Hospital for Joint Diseases*, **72**, 164.

Kahn RL, Stanton MA, Tong-Ngork S, *et al.* (2008) One-year experience with day-of-surgery pregnancy testing before elective orthopedic procedures. *Anesthesia and Analgesia*, **106**, 1127.

Kraft WK, Adeniyi-Jones SC, Chervoneva I, *et al.* (2017) Buprenorphine for the treatment of the neonatal abstinence syndrome. *New England Journal of Medicine*, **376**, 2341.

Ling W, Mooney L, and Torrington M. (2012) Buprenorphine for opioid addiction. *Pain Management*, **2**, 345.

Manley S, de Kelaita G, Joseph NJ, *et al.* (1995) Preoperative pregnancy testing in ambulatory surgery. *Anesthesiology*, **83**, 690.

Mazze RI and Kallen B. (1989) Reproductive outcome after anesthesia and operation during pregnancy: a Registry study of 5405 cases. *American Journal of Obstetrics and Gynecology*, **161**, 1178.

Nezvalová-Henriksen K, Spigset O, and Nordeng H. (2012) Effects of codeine on pregnancy outcome: results from a large population-based cohort study. *European Journal of Clinical Pharmacology*, **68**, 1689.

Pasternak B and Hviid A. (2010) Use of acyclovir, valacyclovir, and famciclovir in the first trimester of pregnancy and the risk of birth defects. *Journal of the American Medical Association*, **304**, 859.

Saxen I. (1975) Associations between oral clefts and drugs taken during pregnancy. *International Journal of Epidemiology*, **4**, 37.

Servey J and Chang J. (2014) Over-the-counter medications in pregnancy. *American Family Physician*, **90**, 548.

Slone D, Shapiro S, and Miettinen O. (1997) Case control surveillance of serious illnesses attributable to ambulatory drug use, in *Epidemiological Evaluation of Drugs* (eds F Colombo, S Shapiro, D Slone, G. Tagnoni), Elsevier/North Holland Biomedical Press, Amsterdam, pp. 59–70.

Stergiakouli E, Thapar A, and Davey Smith G. (2016) Association of acetaminophen use during pregnancy with behavioral problems in childhood: evidence against confounding. *JAMA Pediatrics*, **170**, 964.

Twersky RS and Singleton G. (1996) Preoperative pregnancy testing: justice and testing for all. *Anesthesia and Analgesia*, **83**, 438.

Yefet E, Salim R, Chazan B, *et al.* (2014) The safety of quinolones in pregnancy. *Obstetrics and Gynecology Survey*, **11**, 681.

Further Reading

Abdallah C. (2011) Teen pregnancy testing. risk documentation versus cancellation? *Journal of Pediatric and Adolescent Gynecology*, **24**, e45.

American College of Obstetricians and Gynecologists (2005) Committee Opinion No. 326. Inappropriate Use of the Terms Fetal Distress and Birth Asphyxia. *Obstetrics and Gynecology*, **106**, 1469.

American College of Obstetricians and Gynecologists. (2011) *Committee Opinion 497. Methamphetamine Abuse in Women of Reproductive Age*. Available online at: https://www.acog.org/Resources-And-Publications/Committee-Opinions/Committee-on-Health-Care-for-Underserved-Women/Methamphetamine-Abuse-in-Women-of-Reproductive-Age (accessed 19 October 2017).

American College of Obstetricians and Gynecologists (2017) Committee Opinion No. 696. Non-Obstetric Surgery During Pregnancy. *Obstetrics and Gynecology*, **129**, 777.

Babb M, Koren G, and Einarson A. (2010) Treating pain during pregnancy. *Canadian Family Physician*, **56**, 25.

Beale DJ. (2017) Acetaminophen in pregnancy and adverse childhood neurodevelopment. *JAMA Pediatrics*, **171**, 394.

Becker DE and Reed KL. (2012) Local anesthetics. Review of pharmacological considerations. *Anesthesia Progress*, **59**, 90.

Bellantuono C, Tofani S, di Sciascio G, *et al.* (2013) Benzodiazepine exposure in pregnancy and risk of major malformations. A critical overview. *General Hospital Psychiatry*, **35**, 3.

Bodin SG, Edwards AF, and Roy RC. (2010) False confidences in preoperative pregnancy testing. *Anesthesia and Analgesia*, **110**, 256.

Bookstaver PB, Bland CM, Griffin B, *et al.* (2015) A review of antibiotic use in pregnancy. *Pharmacotherapy*, **35**, 1052.

Bural GG, Laymon CM, and Mountz JM. (2012) Nuclear imaging of a pregnant patient. Should we perform nuclear medicine procedures during pregnancy? *MIRT*, **21**, 1.

Cannabis in the United States. Available online at: https:/ en.wikipedia.org/ wiki/ Cannabis_in_the_United_States

Cengiz SB. (2007) The dental patient. Considerations for dental management and drug use. *Quintessence International*, **38**, 133.

Chen MM, Coakley FV, Kaimal A, *et al.* (2008) Guidelines for computed tomography and magnetic resonance imaging use during pregnancy and lactation. *Obstetrics and Gynecology*, **112**, 333.

Cleves MA, Savell VH Jr, Raj S, *et al.* (2004) Maternal use of acetaminophen and nonsteroidal anti-inflammatory drugs (NSAIDs), and muscular ventricular septal defects. *Birth Defects Research A Clinical and Molecular Teratology*, **70**, 107.

Coakley F, Gould R, Hess C, *et al. Guidelines for the Use of CT and MRI During Pregnancy and Lactation.* Available online at: https:// radiology.ucsf.edu/patient-care/patient-safety/ct-mri-pregnancy (accessed 19 October 2017).

Colgan L, Cook VA, Currie WJR, *et al.* (2011) Recording of pregnancy status before surgery. *British Journal of Oral and Maxillofacial Surgery*, **49S**, S44.

Council on Clinical Affairs (2015) Guideline on use of local anesthesia for pediatric dental patient. *American Academy of Pediatric Dentistry*, **38**, 204.

D'Amore MM, Cheng DM, Kressin NR, *et al.* (2011) Oral health of substance-dependent individuals. *Impact of specific substances. Journal of Substance Abuse Treatment*, **41**, 179.

Dawkins L and Concoran O. (2014) Acute electronic cigarette use. nicotine delivery and subjective effects in regular users. *Psychopharmacology*, **231**, 401.

Dellinger TM and Livingston MH. (2006) Pregnancy. Physiologic changes and considerations for dental patients. *Dental Clinics of North America*, **50**, 677.

Dempsey D and Benowitz L. (2001) Risks and benefits of nicotine to aid smoking cessation in pregnancy. *Drug Safety*, **24**, 277.

Doheny K. (2016) *Acetaminophen and Pregnancy. Bad Mix?* Available online at: https://www.webmd.com/baby/ news/20160817/acetaminophen-pregnancy-bad-mix#1 (accessed 19 October 2017).

Donaldson M and Goodchild JH. (2012) Pregnancy, breast-feeding and drugs used in dentistry. *Journal of the American Dental Association*, **143**, 858.

Duncan PG and Pope WDB. (1996) Medical ethics and legal standards. *Anesthesia and Analgesia*, **82**, 1.

Duncan PG, Pope WDB, Cohen MM, *et al.* (1986) Fetal risk of anesthesia and surgery during pregnancy. *Anesthesiology*, **64**, 790.

Etter JF, Zather E, and Svensson S. (2013) Analysis of refill liquids for electronic cigarettes. *Addiction*, **10**, 1.

Farquhar B, Mark K, Terplan M, *et al.* (2015) Demystifying electronic cigarette use in pregnancy. *Journal of Addiction Medicine*, **9**, 157.

Fayans EP, Stuart HR, Carsten D, *et al.* (2010) Local anesthetic use in the pregnant and postpartum patient. *Dental Clinics of North America*, **54**, 697.

Flynn TR and Susarla SM. (2007) Oral and maxillofacial surgery for the pregnant patient. *Oral and Maxillofacial Surgical Clinics of North America*, **19**, 207.

Gin T. (1994) Propofol during pregnancy. *Acta Anaesthesiologica Sinica*, **32**, 127.

Gravett C, Eckert LO, and Gravett MG. (2016) Non-reassuring fetal status. Case definition and guidelines for data collection, analysis, and presentation of immunization safety data. *Vaccine*, **34**, 6084.

Guay J. (2009) Methemoglobinemia related to local anesthetics. A summary of 242 episodes. *Anesthesia and Analgesia*, **108**, 837.

Gupta P and Subramoney S. (2004) Smokeless tobacco use, birth weight, and gestational age. population based, prospective cohort study of 1217 women in Mumbai, India. *British Medical Journal*, **328**, 1538.

Gurney J, Richiardi L, McGlynn KA, *et al.* (2017) Analgesia use during pregnancy and risk of cryptorchidism. a systematic review and meta-analysis. *Human Reproduction*, **32**, 1118.

Hutzler C, Paschke M, Kruschinski S, *et al.* (2014) Chemical hazards present in liquids and vapors of electronic cigarettes. *Archives of Toxicology*, **88**, 1295.

Jensen RP, Wentai L, Pankow JF, *et al.* (2015) Formaldehyde in E-cigarette aerosols. *New England Journal of Medicine*, **372**, 392.

Jones TB, Bailey BA, and Sokol RJ. (2013) Alcohol use in pregnancy. Insights in screening and intervention for the clinician. *Clinical Obstetrics and Gynecology*, **56**, 114.

Kanal E, Shellock FG, and Talagala L. (1990) Safety considerations in MR imaging. *Radiology*, **176**, 593–606.

Kang SH, Chua-Gocheco A, Bozzo P, *et al.* (2011) Safety of antiviral medication for the treatment of herpes during pregnancy. *Canadian Family Physician*, **57**, 427.

Kemp MW, Newnham JP, Challis JG, *et al.* (2016) The clinical use of corticosteroids in pregnancy. *Human Reproduction Update*, **22**, 240.

Khan I, Ansari MI, and Khan R. (2010) Oral surgery for the pregnant patient. *Heal Talk*, **3**, 31.

Kieser JA, Groeneveld HT, and da Silva CF. (1997) Dental asymmetry, maternal obesity, and smoking. *American Journal of Physical Anthropology*, **102**, 133.

Kim HJ and Shin HS. (2013) Determination of tobacco-specific nitrosamines in replacement liquids of electronic cigarettes by liquid chromatography-tandem mass spectrometry. *Journal of Chromatography*, **1291**, 48.

Ko H, Kaye AD, and Urman RD. (2014) Nitrous oxide and perioperative outcomes. *Journal of Anesthesia*, **28**, 420.

Kurien S, Kattimani VS, Sriram RR, *et al.* (2013) Management of pregnant patient in dentistry. *Journal of International Oral Health*, **5**, 88.

Maher JL and Mahabir RC. (2012) Preoperative pregnancy testing. *Canadian Journal of Plastic Surgery*, **20**, e32.

Malaika B, Koren G, and Einarson A. (2010) Treating pain during pregnancy. *Canadian Family Physician*, **56**, 25.

Mallikarjuna R and Nalawade T. (2014) Alcohol, its effect on dental structures and the role of a dentist. *Journal of Alcohol and Drug Dependence*, **2**, 4.

Mandim BLS. (2015) Review of anesthesia for non-obstetrical surgery during pregnancy. *Journal of Community Medicine and Health Education*, **5**, 346.

Mavrogenis S, Urban R, Czeizel AE, *et al.* (2014) Maternal risk factors in the origin of isolated hypospadias – a population-based case–control study. *Congenital Anomalies*, **54**, 110.

McDonnell-Naughton M, McGarvey C, O'Regan M, *et al.* (2012) Maternal smoking and alcohol consumption during pregnancy as risk factors for sudden infant death. *Irish Medical Journal*, **105**, 105–108.

McQueen KA, Murphy-Oikonen J, and Desaulniers L. (2015) Maternal substance use and neonatal abstinence syndrome. A descriptive study. *Maternal and Child Health Journal*, **19**, 1756.

Merritt TA, Wilkinson B, and Chervenak C. (2016) Maternal use of marijuana during pregnancy and lactation. Implications for infant and child development and their well-being. *Academic Journal of Pediatrics and Neonatology*, **2**, 1.

Meyer KD and Zhang L. (2009) Short- and long-term adverse effects of cocaine abuse during pregnancy on the heart development. *Therapeutic Advances in Cardiovascular Disease*, **3**, 7.

Moon TS and Sappenfield J. (2016) Anesthetic management and challenges in the pregnant patient. *Current Anesthesiology Reports*, **6**, 89.

Naseem M, Khurshid Z, Khan HA, *et al.* (2016) Oral health challenges in pregnant women. Recommendations for dental care professionals. *Saudi Journal of Dental Research*, **7**, 138.

National Institute for Occupational Safety and Health (NIOSH) *Control of Nitrous Oxide in Dental Operatories* (DHHS/NIOSH Publication No. 96-107). Available online at: www.cdc.gov/niosh/docs/hazardcontrol/hc3.html (accessed 19 October 2017).

National Institute on Drug Abuse (2014) *Heroin*. Available online at: www.drugabuse.gov/publications/research-reports/heroin (accessed 19 October 2017).

Neuman G and Koren G. (2013) Safety of procedural sedation in pregnancy. *Journal of Obstetrics and Gynaecology Canada*, **35**, 168.

Ouanounou A and Haas DA. (2016) Drug therapy during pregnancy. Implications for dental practice. *British Dental Journal*, **220**, 413.

Pacifici GM. (2006) Placental transfer of antibiotics administered to the mother. A review. *International Journal of Clinical Pharmacology and Therapeutics*, **44**, 57.

Peters SL, Lind JN, and Humphrey JR. (2013) Safe lists for medications in pregnancy. Inadequate evidence base and inconsistent guidance from Web-based information, 2011. *Pharmacoepidemiology and Drug Safety*, **22**, 324–328.

Pilmis B, Jullien V, Sobel J, *et al.* (2015) Antifungal drugs during pregnancy. An updated review. *Journal of Antimicrobial Chemotherapy*, **70**, 14.

Reitman E and Flood P. (2011) Anaesthetic considerations for non-obstetric surgery during pregnancy. *British Journal of Anaesthesia*, **107**, i72.

Schweitzer A. (2006) Dietary supplements during pregnancy. *Journal of Perinatal Education*, **15**, 44.

Shekarchizadeh H, Khami MR, and Mohebbi SZ. (2013) Oral health of drug abusers. A review of health effects and care. *Iranian Journal of Public Health*, **42**, 929.

Shessel BA, Portnof JE, Kaltman SI, *et al.* (2013) Dental treatment of the pregnant patient. Literature review and guidelines for the practicing clinician. *Today's FDA*, **25**, 26–29.

Shetty L, Shete A, and Gupta AA. (2015) Pregnant oral and maxillofacial patient – Catch 22 situation. *Dentistry*, **5**, 9.

Shetty V, Harrell L, Murphy DA, *et al.* (2015) Dental disease patterns in methamphetamine users. Findings in a large urban sample. *Journal of the American Dental Association*, **146**, 875.

Singer LT, Moore DG, Min MO, *et al.* (2012) One-year outcomes of prenatal exposure to MDMA and other recreational drugs. *Pediatrics*, **130**, 407.

Soraisham AS. (2016) Maternal codeine and its effect on the fetus and neonate. A focus on pharmacogenomics, neuropathology, and withdrawal, in *Neuropathology of Drug Addictions and Substance Misuse*, vol. 3 (ed. VR Preedy), Academic Press, New York, pp. 392–397.

Takalkar AM, Khandelwal A, Lokitz S, *et al.* (2011) 18 F-FDG PET in pregnancy and fetal radiation dose estimates. *Journal of Nuclear Medicine*, **52**, 1035.

Tanaka K, Miyake Y, and Sasaki S. (2009) The effect of maternal smoking during pregnancy and postnatal household smoking on dental caries in young children. *Journal of Pediatrics*, **155**, 410.

Turner M and Aziz SR. (2002) Management of the pregnant oral and maxillofacial surgery patient. *Journal of Oral and Maxillofacial Surgery*, **60**, 1479.

Upadya M and Saneesh PJ. (2016) Anaesthesia for non-obstetric surgery during pregnancy. *Indian Journal of Anaesthesia*, **60**, 234.

Wang P, Chong S, Kielar A, *et al.* (2012) Imaging of pregnant and lactating patients. Part 1, Evidence-based review and recommendations. *American Journal of Roentgenology*, **198**, 778.

Ward RK and Zamorski MA. (2002) Benefits and risks of psychiatric medications during pregnancy. *American Family Physician*, **66**, 629.

Wendell AD. (2013) Overview and epidemiology of substance abuse in pregnancy. *Clinical Obstetrics and Gynecology*, **56**, 91.

Werler MM. (2006) Teratogen update. Pseudoephedrine. *Birth Defects Research A Clinical and Molecular Teratology*, **76**, 445.

Wikstrom A, Cnattingius S, and Stephansson O. (2010) Maternal use of Swedish snuff (snus) and risk of stillbirth. *Epidemiology*, **21**, 772.

Wilkening RB and Meschia G. (1983) Fetal oxygen uptake, oxygenation, and acid–base balance as a function of uterine blood flow. *American Journal of Physiology – Heart and Circulatory Physiology*, **244**, H749.

Wingfield M and McMenamin M. (2014) Preoperative pregnancy testing. *British Journal of Surgery*, **101**, 1488.

Women's Health Series (2000) Herbs of special interest to women. *Journal of the American Pharmacists' Association*, **40**, 234.

Yau WP, Mitchel AA, Lin KJ, *et al.* (2013) Use of decongestants during pregnancy and the risk of birth defects. *American Journal of Epidemiology*, **178**, 198.

Yazdy MM, Desai RJ, and Brogly SB. (2015) Prescription opioids in pregnancy and birth outcomes. A review of the literature. *Journal of Pediatric Genetics*, **4**, 56.

5

Dental and Oral Diseases in Pregnancy

Christos A. Skouteris

Prenatal Counseling and Prevention

Pregnancy is a time when women can be motivated to adopt healthy behavior. This is also an opportune time for pregnant women to learn about practices that promote oral health. It is incumbent upon health providers to educate pregnant women about the impact of good oral health on the well-being of the mother and fetus. Statistics have shown that 56% of women do not have any dental care during pregnancy and that 59% of pregnant women do not receive any counseling on oral health issues. Factors contributing to these statistics include the possibility that ob-gyn providers do not routinely incorporate oral health discussions into their clinical practices, and the fact that some dental providers avoid treating pregnant women because of confusion and misconceptions about the safety and importance of dental treatment during pregnancy. Additional compounding factors include the inability to access dental care by low-income and underprivileged women.

Prenatal oral health counseling is very important in informing the pregnant woman on the risks that poor oral health poses for the mother and fetus. These risks include the following.

- Vertical transmission of cariogenic *Streptococcus mutans* (*S. mutans*) from the mother to the infant, with a significant risk for future caries experience and potentially low infant birth weight.
- *Preterm birth*: although an evidence-based cause-and-effect relationship between high maternal *S. mutans*/caries/periodontal disease and preterm births has not been established yet, some indication exists in the literature for their potential association.
- *Fetal growth restriction*: circulating inflammatory mediators (such as cytokines, prostaglandins, interleukins, tumor necrosis factor, and endotoxins) resulting from periodontal disease have been incriminated as a potential cause of preterm births and restriction of fetal growth.
- Severe and even life-threatening odontogenic infections.

Strategies that should be implemented to provide effective oral health prenatal counseling should include the following.

- Educating the pregnant woman about the importance of oral health as it relates to her health and that of her children.
- Encouraging and assisting pregnant women in seeking dental care during pregnancy, especially if they have oral health problems
- Providing and reinforcing messages about how to achieve and maintain good oral health.

Dental Management of the Pregnant Patient, First Edition. Edited by Christos A. Skouteris.
© 2018 John Wiley & Sons, Inc. Published 2018 by John Wiley & Sons, Inc.

- Educating the mother about good oral health practices for the infant that help in reducing the risk of caries.
- Assuring the mother that dental care is safe and effective throughout the pregnancy.
- Educating the mother or caregiver about behaviors that assist in the transmission of cariogenic bacteria through saliva sharing.

Prenatal oral counseling is part of the national consensus for the provision of oral health care during pregnancy which encompasses the following general guidelines for dental professionals.

- Assess pregnant women's oral health.
- Advise pregnant women about oral healthcare.
- Work in collaboration with prenatal care health professionals.
- Provide oral disease management and treatment to pregnant women.
- Provide support services (case management) to pregnant women (assist pregnant women in seeking insurance or other coverage, social services, or other needs; facilitate referrals to prenatal care health professionals in the community).
- Improve health services in the community (establish partnerships with community-based programs that support pregnant women; provide referral to a nutrition professional; provide culturally and linguistically appropriate care).

For more information, the reader is referred to *Oral Health Care During Pregnancy: A National Consensus Statement* published by the National Maternal and Child Health Resource Center, available at: www.mchoralhealth.org.

In recognition of the importance of prenatal oral health counseling, the American College of Obstetricians and Gynecologists in cooperation with the American Dental Association formulated the following recommendations for obstetrician-gynecologists who are for many women the most frequently accessed healthcare professional.

- Discuss oral health with all patients, including those who are pregnant or in the postpartum period.
- Advise women that oral healthcare improves a woman's general health throughout her lifespan and may also reduce the transmission of potentially caries-producing oral bacteria from mothers to their infants.
- Conduct an oral health assessment during the first prenatal visit.
- Reassure patients that prevention, diagnosis, and treatment of oral conditions, including dental X-rays (with shielding of the abdomen and thyroid) and local anesthesia (lidocaine with or without epinephrine), are safe during pregnancy.
- Inform women that conditions that require immediate treatment, such as extractions, root canals, and restorations (amalgam or composite) of untreated caries, may be managed at any time during pregnancy. Delaying treatment may result in more complex problems.
- For patients with vomiting secondary to morning sickness, hyperemesis gravidarum, or gastric reflux during late pregnancy, the use of antacids or rinsing with a baking soda solution (i.e., one teaspoon of baking soda dissolved in one cup of water) may help neutralize the associated acid.
- Be aware of patients' health coverage for dental services during pregnancy so that referrals to the appropriate dental provider can be made. Note that each state's Medicaid coverage for oral health may vary considerably.
- Develop a working relationship with local dentists. Refer patients for oral healthcare with a written note or call, as would be the practice with referrals to any medical specialist.
- Advocate the broader oral health coverage of women before, during, and after pregnancy. Pregnancy is a unique time when women may gain access to oral health coverage.

- Reinforce routine oral health maintenance, such as limiting sugary foods and drinks, brushing twice a day with fluoridated toothpaste, flossing once daily, and dental visits twice a year.

Note: Currently, there are no studies regarding the teratogenic potential of fluoride supplements. Additionally, there is no proof of efficacy. Therefore, fluoride supplements cannot be recommended. There is no evidence that fluoride in the drinking water or in toothpaste poses a health risk to the fetus *in utero* or postpartum.

Further Reading

American College of Obstetricians and Gynecologists (2013) Committee Opinion 569. Oral health care during pregnancy and throughout the lifespan. *Obstetrics and Gynecology*, **122**, 417.

Connecticut State Dental Association (2013) *Considerations for the Dental Treatment of Pregnant Women: A Resource for Connecticut Dentists*. Connecticut State Dental Association with assistance from the Connecticut Section of the American College of Obstetricians and Gynecologists and the Connecticut Chapter of the American Academy of Family Physicians, Connecticut.

Leverett DH, Adair SM, Vaughan BW, *et al.* (1997) Randomized clinical trial of the effect of prenatal fluoride supplements in preventing dental caries. *Caries Research*, **31**, 174.

Maturo P, Costacurta M, Perugia C, *et al.* (2011) Fluoride supplements in pregnancy: effectiveness in the prevention of dental caries in a group of children. *Oral Implantology* **4**, 23.

Michigan Department of Health and Human Services (2015) *During Pregnancy the Mouth Matters: A Guide to Michigan Perinatal Oral Health*. Michigan Department of Health and Human Services in association with Delta Dental of Michigan, Lansing, Michigan, pp. 7–9.

National Maternal and Child Oral Health Resource Center (2012) Oral Health Care During Pregnancy: A National Consensus Statement. National Maternal and Child Oral Health Resource Center, Washington DC, pp. 4–5.

Vamos CA, Walsh ML, Thompson E, *et al.* (2015) Oral-systemic health during pregnancy: exploring prenatal and oral health providers' information, motivation and behavioral skills. *Maternal and Child Health Journal*, **19**, 1263.

6

Dental, Oral, and Maxillofacial Diseases and Conditions and Their Treatment

Treatment of Dental Disease

Benjamin Craig Cornwall

Very often dentists have to face a pregnant woman's anxiety – along with her family's anxiety – over the matter of the safety of dental treatment during pregnancy. This is due to a series of wrong assumptions that have been perpetuated by the lack of proper information, as well as by some dental professionals who consider dental treatments to be possibly dangerous for the fetus. It is highly unlikely any dental procedure would induce spontaneous abortion. However, febrile illness and sepsis can. It is beyond doubt that dental treatment during pregnancy is not only safe but also necessary. Dental care has been proven to be not only safe and effective during pregnancy but also necessary to promote sound oral health. It is imperative that dental treatment be coordinated among obstetric and oral healthcare providers. During pregnancy, dental treatment may be modified but need not be withheld, provided that the risk assessment is made properly for both the patient and the fetus.

Although there has been improvement in the dental care of pregnant women during the past decades, inequalities and erroneous perceptions concerning the importance of dental care during pregnancy still exist, affecting mainly the socioeconomically deprived in the population. Many organizations, including the American Dental Association (ADA), the

American Academy of Pediatrics (AAP), and the American Academy of Pediatric Dentistry (AAPD), have developed protocols and norms in order to improve the oral health of pregnant women and babies. They stress that pregnancy is not a disease, so pregnant women should not be treated differently from the general population. Still, the dentist needs to be aware of the altered physiologic status of the pregnant patient to avoid inappropriate interpretation of normal changes in physiology (see Chapter 2). Pregnancy by itself is not a reason to defer routine dental care or necessary dental treatment. However, prudence may dictate that elective treatment is deferred until after delivery.

Questionnaire

During the initial visit or during a return visit with a pregnant patient, a thorough questionnaire needs to be completed or updated. While your questionnaire should be in depth, some additional information needs to be compiled.

Patient

What trimester, recent changes in BP – specifically new-onset HTN, previous miscarriages, recent cramping/Braxton-Hicks contractions (see Chapter 9), any bleeding/spotting, any intraoral changes (newly developed lesions, bleeding gums?), name and address and contact information of OB/GYN.

Dental Management of the Pregnant Patient, First Edition. Edited by Christos A. Skouteris.
© 2018 John Wiley & Sons, Inc. Published 2018 by John Wiley & Sons, Inc.

To complete the information required to treat the patient some additional information from the OB/GYN is needed.

OB/GYN

The following items should be addressed by obtaining a medical consultation.

- Treatment of any preexisting past medical conditions (aside from pregnancy) (e.g., hypertension, diabetes, heparin intake).
- Clarification of all medications being provided to the patient during pregnancy.
- Any specific restrictions on meds, radiographs.
- High-risk pregnancy?
- Expected delivery date.
- Discussion of medical complications that may be the result of pregnancy.
- Any special treatment recommendations that may improve individualized care for the pregnant patient.

Dental Examination

As with the questionnaire, the dental examination needs to be complete. The elements of the exam are well documented. The completeness of this exam, as with all exams, is that it is comprehensive.

The major topics that need to be addressed in both the medical interview and dental examination include the following.

- HPI/Current problem list
- Medical history
- Surgical history
- Dental history
- Clinical evaluation: intraoral examination
- Extraoral examination
- Dental examination
- Periodontal examination
- Radiographic examination
- Oral health instruction (OHI)

Provided that the pregnant woman is healthy, a dentist does not normally need the obstetrician's consent in order to perform common dental procedures. However, if for some reason the dentist thinks that the dental treatment should be postponed or if there are any comorbid conditions for which the patient receives medication that may affect dental treatment, the dentist should inform and consult the obstetrician.

Similarly, the obstetrician should be informed if the dentist thinks it necessary that the pregnant woman should be treated in a hospital setting, especially if the dental treatment should be performed under general anesthesia. A dentist is critical to the medical care of his/her patients. Often, by attention to the health status of the patient, the OB/GYN can be advised of changes in the medical condition that may warrant follow-up.

Special Considerations

There are a number of issues unique to pregnancy that will affect whether the patient can receive dental care. Often, especially as the pregnancy progresses, there will be an increase in the need to urinate as the bladder is compressed. When treating patients, this will affect timing and length of procedures. Additionally, especially in the first trimester, patients tend to be nauseous and develop an aversion to smells. As is common knowledge, the dental treatment room often has a unique smell to it. This may stimulate your patient in a negative manner. Then, there is the potential for an increased gag reflex. The ability to have dental instruments in the mouth and even tolerate impressions may be greatly reduced. Finally, there is an alteration in taste. Previously acceptable tastes may no longer be tolerated. All of this can affect dental treatment.

There is also a concern regarding an increase in appetite. Patients are often snacking throughout the day – the cravings of legend. As is well established, frequency of exposure to fermentable sugars is more significant than total amounts. There is the very real risk of increased caries in patients with little to no previous risk and an exacerbation of risk in previously high-risk patients. With the previously mentioned problems associated with pregnant patients, treatment can become a challenge. This all places greater importance on OHI. An emphasis on good home care as well as seeking professional care is paramount.

Common Conditions and Their Treatment

Pregnancy Gingivitis

Pregnancy gingivitis is considered the most common oral manifestation of pregnancy and has been reported as occurring in up to 100% of pregnant women.

Pregnancy gingivitis commonly becomes apparent later in the second month of gestation and worsens as the pregnancy progresses before reaching a peak in the eighth month. In the last month of gestation, gingivitis usually decreases and immediately post partum the gingival tissues are found to be comparable to those seen during the second month of gestation.

Increased erythema, edema, and bleeding are thought to be the result of increased levels of progesterone and effects on microvascularity since progesterone and estradiol stimulate prostaglandin synthesis in the gingival tissues.

Management of pregnancy gingivitis involves regular dental visits for professional cleaning and monitoring with education of the woman regarding both the etiology and prevention of the condition.

Periodontal Disease

Because infections (such as urinary tract infection) in pregnant women are associated with preterm birth and low birth weight, the hypothesis has been formulated that periodontitis is possibly linked to preterm birth. This hypothesis was supported by experiments that showed fetal growth restriction in pregnant women who were affected by periodontitis. The hypothesis is that periodontal pathogens, mainly those belonging to the group of Gram-negative anaerobic rods, affect fetal growth either through their toxins or through the release of inflammatory mediators. This hypothesis has been explored in numerous scientific publications.

Although the causal role of specific bacteria in pregnancy-associated gingivitis has been difficult to establish, gingival bleeding and inflammation appear to be associated with a rise in the numbers of Gram-negative rods present. However, an increase in the selective growth of *Porphyromonas* (*P. intermedia*, *P. gingivalis* – formerly *Bacteroides*) and *Tannerella* species has been demonstrated in subgingival plaque during the onset of pregnancy gingivitis. This is likely to be a result of these species being able to use the pregnancy hormones, particularly progesterone, as a source of nutrition. This increase in selective growth may also be favored by the changes that occur in the immune system during pregnancy alongside those that develop locally in the gingival crevice, such as blood from bleeding gingiva providing further nutrients and increased pocket depths creating a more favorable environment for anaerobes.

Not all studies have found an association between periodontal disease and preterm delivery and low birth weight. So far, the results of these studies have been conflicting as, according to some researchers, it has been estimated that periodontal treatment in pregnant women has not reduced the risk of preterm low birth-weight infants whereas others report positive results regarding the prevention of such occurrences. One study found that the risk actually decreased with increasing pocket depth. Another study found no association between periodontal disease and preterm delivery and low birth weight, although, interestingly, this work did suggest a link between indicators of poor periodontal health and late miscarriage.

Recently, a systematic review concluded that periodontal disease may be adversely associated with pregnancy outcome. Recent research has suggested that pregnant women who received successful periodontal treatment based on strict criteria had a significantly lower risk of undergoing preterm labor. The same research suggested that the hormonal state of pregnant women makes periodontal therapy more challenging. Bearing all of this in mind, it is hoped that current research, in particular interventional studies on pregnant women with periodontal disease, may help to establish whether a significant cause-and-effect relationship does exist and the impact periodontal treatment may have during pregnancy. Additionally, there should be more studies that focus not only on the periodontal treatment procedure, but also on its success as well as the time that the treatment takes place.

The point to be taken from the above is that there is an association with periodontal disease and preterm low birth weight, but no causal relationship has been established. Maternal periodontitis is modestly but not independently associated with adverse pregnancy outcomes. This does not mean that an adequate oral health maintenance program is not important. Even with all of these contradictory findings, it is important to remember that periodontal therapy in general, and scaling and root planing in particular, are safe and appropriate if indicated. Furthermore, one must always be aware that gestational diabetes increases the risk of periodontal disease.

Attrition/Tooth Surface Loss

Tooth surface loss, primarily through acid-induced erosion, may be seen if there has been nausea and associated repeated vomiting during pregnancy. The palatal surfaces of the maxillary incisors and canines are often the most affected. The patient commonly presents complaining of sensitivity, which is a consequence of the resulting dentine exposure. Management is essentially preventive and includes the regular use of a fluoride mouth rinse, especially in those women with hyperemesis gravidarum and gastric reflux. In addition, these women should be advised to avoid tooth brushing directly after vomiting as the effect of erosion can be exacerbated by brushing an already demineralized tooth surface.

Halitosis

There are many contributing conditions to the development or worsening of halitosis during pregnancy. In addition to poor oral hygiene in general and other factors such as smoking, alcohol, and substance abuse during pregnancy, these conditions include:

- hormonal changes (e.g., pregnancy gingivitis)
- periodontal disease
- caries
- xerostomia
- oral candidiasis
- oral mucosal lesions (e.g., pemhigoid gestationis)
- vomiting, hyperemesis gravidarum
- gastric reflux
- altered eating habits
- gestational diabetes.

Treatment is aimed at addressing as many of these conditions as possible by managing dental caries and periodontal disease, treating oral candidiasis and mucosal lesions, advocating good hydration and use of oral moisturizers, recommending the use of antacids and soda mouth rinses, advising on proper dietary adaptations, encouraging frequent dental visits, and reinforcing the importance of maintaining good oral hygiene.

Tooth Mobility

Increased tooth mobility has been detected in pregnancy, even in periodontally healthy women. The upper incisors are most mobile during the last month of pregnancy. Development of such mobility is possibly due to mineral shifts in the lamina dura and not to modification of the alveolar bone as there is often no apparent loss of bone support noted on radiographic evaluation. The degree of periodontal disease present and disturbance of the supporting attachment tissues are also thought to contribute to this mobility, which usually resolves post partum. There is no evidence of a need for additional calcium supplements and treatment is symptomatic and only as required.

Caries

The dietary changes that may occur, especially in early pregnancy, such as regular consumption of sugary snacks and drinks to satisfy cravings or to prevent nausea and sickness, will result in an increased risk of dental caries unless extra attention is paid to oral hygiene. This can be further complicated if the pregnant woman is unable to tolerate tooth brushing because of nausea and sickness to the extent that tooth brushing is significantly compromised.

The treatment required consists of treating the dental caries and emphasizing improved home and professional dental care. Caries has to be effectively managed to avoid the potential complications from tooth decay, with the most important being acute or chronic severe odontalgia and infection. Endodontic treatment in pregnancy should be part of the overall management of dental caries. It has been asserted that neither the cleansing irrigant hypochlorite nor root canal filling materials used in endodontic treatment are detrimental to the fetus.

Timing of Dental Treatment

Traditionally, dental treatment of any kind has been avoided during the first trimester of pregnancy, so as not to harm the fetus during organogenesis. However, there is not enough evidence to forbid dental treatment even during the first trimester of pregnancy. Emergency dental procedures are indicated at all times during pregnancy and can be performed during any trimester when a delay in necessary treatment could result in significant risk to the mother and an indirect risk to the fetus. Special precautions may be needed during these instances.

For elective dental procedures, the ideal period for complete dental treatment of a pregnant woman is the beginning of the second trimester (14–20 weeks of pregnancy). At this stage, there is no risk of teratogenesis, nausea and vomiting have subsided, and the uterus is not yet large enough to cause discomfort. However, it is important to

remember that extensive reconstruction, crown and bridge as well as removable partial dentures should be deferred until after pregnancy.

First Trimester (Box 6.1)

The time generally accepted for the first trimester ranges from the first day of the last menstrual period until 13 weeks and 6 days of gestation. Within this time frame, it is important to remember that the period from 2 to 4 weeks from the last menstrual period represents the predifferentiation period of the fetus. During this period, the fetus is relatively resistant to teratogens. The period of greatest teratogenic risk is organogenesis, the time at which the fetus is most susceptible to malformation, which occurs from the end of the predifferentiation period to the end of the 10th week after the last menstrual period.

Second Trimester (Box 6.2)

The second trimester comprises weeks 14–27 of gestation. During this period, the fetus undergoes growth and maturation. The important thing to remember is that during this trimester, the teeth are forming and are susceptible to malformation. It is generally accepted that it is best to defer elective treatment to the second trimester and first half of the third trimester. The goal here is controlling

---

Box 6.1 First trimester – recommendations.

- Educate the patient about maternal oral changes during pregnancy
- Emphasize strict oral hygiene instructions and thereby plaque control
- Limit dental treatment to periodontal prophylaxis and emergency treatments only
- Avoid elective procedures
- Avoid routine radiographs. Use selectively and when needed
- This is the most likely time you will find it necessary to consult with the patient's physician

> **Box 6.2 Second trimester –
> recommendations.**
>
> - Oral hygiene instruction and plaque control
> - Scaling, polishing, and curettage may be performed if necessary
> - Control of active oral diseases, if any
> - Elective dental care is safe (root canals, extractions, restorations)
> - Avoid routine radiographs. Use selectively and when needed

active disease and eliminating potential problems for the remainder of the pregnancy and immediately post partum. You want to avoid extensive restorations and comprehensive treatment.

Third Trimester (Box 6.3)

The third trimester runs from 28 weeks gestation until birth. Beginning after the first half of the third trimester, you want to avoid elective procedures. The concern at this point of the pregnancy is maternal comfort. Appointments greater than 30 minutes tend to compound the problem. Pressure on the bladder can increase urinary urgency and there is a very real risk of supine hypotensive syndrome.

Dental Materials and Their Significance in Pregnancy

Exposure to mercury and acrylate compounds occurs during the placement and removal of amalgam or composite restorations,

> **Box 6.3 Third trimester –
> recommendations.**
>
> - Oral hygiene instruction and plaque control
> - Scaling, polishing, and curettage may be performed if necessary
> - Active oral diseases should be controlled
> - Radiograph use should be minimized
> - It's safe to perform elective procedures, but avoid elective dental care during the second half of the third trimester

the finishing and polishing of restorations, and throughout the lifespan of the restoration. The use of amalgam in dentistry has decreased during the past decade, whereas the use of composites consisting of methacrylic compounds has increased. When a restoration is required during pregnancy, the patient needs to be informed of the different options, and, together with the dentist, they should decide on the best material to use. Using a rubber dam and high-speed evacuation (suction) during amalgam or composite placement and/or removal may significantly reduce the inhalation of mercury elements (mercury vapor) and acrylate compounds. Unfortunately, once there is a need to restore a tooth due to caries, it is very difficult to avoid potentially harmful materials, with the possible exception of cohesive gold foil.

Amalgam

Dental amalgam has been a restorative material of choice for around 175 years. The potential toxic effects have been known for around 150 years. There is a great deal of misconception associated with the controversy regarding the safety of this material.

Inorganic mercury in three different forms and methylated mercury all have different absorption pathways and their metabolism and storage within the body are different. Mercury is naturally present in the environment. It is impossible for humans to avoid exposure to some form of mercury from the environment. Significantly, however, in addition to environmental exposure, individuals may be exposed to Hg from dental amalgams, medicinal treatments (including vaccinations), as well as dietary sources.

Elemental mercury ($Hg0$) exists as a liquid at room temperature, and because of its high vapor pressure, it is released readily into the atmosphere as Hg vapor. The main source of exposure to inorganic mercury (I-Hg) is dental amalgam restorations, which release $Hg0$. Inorganic mercury also exists in two other forms: mercuric ($Hg2+$) and mercurous ($Hg+$). One route of exposure to $Hg2+$ and $Hg+$ is via food and/or liquids contaminated with Hg2+ and/or Hg+. Methylmercury (CH$_3$Hg+) (MeHg) is by far the most common form of organic mercury to which humans and animals are exposed, primarily from food and most significantly from fish.

Absorption of these forms into the body is also different. Hg0 is absorbed by the lungs. Hg+ and Hg2+ are poorly absorbed by the gut and the methylated forms are more readily absorbed through the intestine. Hg0 in the lungs has a clearance half-life of 29–60 days, but some of it is converted in the lungs to Hg2+ and picked up by the blood. The kidneys are the primary storage site for inorganic mercury while fat storage is the primary site for organic mercury.

Mercuric ions have a high affinity for various nucleophilic groups, in particular the sulfhydryl group that is present in glutathione (GSH), cysteine (Cys), homocysteine (Hcy), N-acetylcysteine (NAC), and albumin. Due to the affinity of these ions for bonding to the reduced sulfur atom, they do not exist as inorganic salts or as unbound, "free" ions. The mercuric ions do not remain bound to these proteins for very long, as evidenced by the rapid decrease in the plasma burden of Hg2+ accompanied by a rapid rate of uptake of mercuric ions in the kidneys, liver, and other organs. The bond with low molecular weight thiols and inorganic mercury is in a linear II coordinate covalent manner. However, the bonding between mercuric ions and these thiol-containing molecules appears to be more labile within the living organism. Organic mercury compounds, such as CH$_3$Hg+, in contrast from linear I coordinate covalent complex with these molecules and are oxidized to Hg2+ by catalase in the blood.

Methylmercury is known to slowly demethylate to inorganic Hg2+ in some tissues; however, the low I-Hg levels found in placentas with high MeHg concentrations seem to indicate negligible demethylation of MeHg in the placenta. Despite the marked placental accumulation of I-Hg, the concentration of I-Hg in umbilical cord blood is similar to that in maternal blood. Most I-Hg likely to be

passed to the fetus is in the form of Hg0. In contrast to the hypothesis that I-Hg is the primary form of Hg that accumulates in the placenta, approximately two-thirds of the Hg stored in placenta is in the form of MeHg.

The concern with the above is the effect on the fetus. It is generally believed that MeHg and Hg0 easily cross the placental barrier whereas Hg2+ is trapped. Inhaled Hg0 is oxidized to inorganic Hg2+ by catalase already within the blood, but small amounts of Hg0 remain in the circulation. The intake and uptake of Hg2+ are negligible. I-Hg (Hg2+ and Hg0) accumulate in the placenta. The median placental concentration is up to four times higher than that in maternal blood and increases with the number of amalgam fillings. Thus, it seems likely that the I-Hg bound in placenta originates from Hg0 released from amalgam restorations.

The amount of mercury vapor released from amalgam restorations (1–10 µg/day) is well below toxic levels. According to the WHO, the total mercury tolerable intake is 2 µg/kg/day. As can be determined from the above, the amount reaching the fetal circulation, while related, is low. Significantly, the ADA, FDA, and WHO consider dental amalgams safe to use in dental restorations, because research has shown that there is no relation between amalgam restorations and complications during pregnancy. Dental amalgam restorations release mercury as a vapor (a form of inorganic mercury) in the mouth and it is well established that levels found are not high enough to produce a teratogenic effect. Additionally, FDA investigations concluded that the fetus/newborn is not at risk from Hg vapors from amalgam *in utero* or from breastfeeding.

Even with the safety of this material established, it is still prudent to practice the safest means of removing and replacing it. The risk of exposure to Hg0 during placement, removal or replacement can be mitigated by the use of a rubber dam and adequate scavenger systems. To minimize the amount of Hg0 that is unbound in the finished restoration, proper technique must be followed.

The amalgam should be well condensed until overfilled and then the mercury-rich layer carved off. When the restoration has initially set, cleaning the surface of the restoration with a moist cotton pellet will remove even more. Finally, consider polishing restorations shortly after placement.

Composites

Resin-based dental materials are composed of organic resins and some other components such as solvents or reinforcing inorganic fillers. The use of composite resin-based restorative materials has increased dramatically over past decades. Other than their obvious esthetic advantages, they have been described as the safe alternative to mercury-based alloys. Early composites used bisphenol A (BPA). Modern composite resins and sealants are formulated from a mixture of monomers that are commonly based on bisphenol A glycidylmethacrylate (Bis-GMA). Some composite resins may contain other monomers, in addition to Bis-GMA, that are added to modify the properties of the resin such as viscosity, handling, and other properties. These monomers include bisphenol A ethoxylate methacrylate (Bis-EMA), bisphenol A dimethacrylate (Bis-DMA), and triethylene glycol dimethacrylate (TEGDMA).

There are two types of BPA derivatives: ones that cannot be hydrolyzed into BPA, such as Bis-GMA and Bis-EMA, and others that can be hydrolyzed into BPA in saliva, such as Bis-DMA. Therefore, even without the presence of BPA directly, BPA can potentially become incorporated into dental composites or sealants in different ways.

- BPA may exist as a byproduct of the degradation of chemical components of resin-based dental materials. Some BPA derivatives with an ester bond (-O-CO-) linking the BPA molecule to the resin, such as Bis-DMA and polycarbonate, have been shown to hydrolyze into BPA. However, the BPA derivatives with ether (-O-) linkage, such as Bis-GMA and Bis-EMA, do not undergo this type of hydrolysis reaction to form BPA.

- BPA may also be found as a trace material, since it may be used in the production of other ingredients found in some dental composites and sealants. Bis-DMA and Bis-GMA are both produced using BPA as a starting ingredient, so residual trace amounts of BPA may be present in the final dental composite or sealant. The amount of BPA from the impurity of BPA derivatives (such as Bis-GMA or Bis-EMA) is usually very low and not detectable (<2 ppm).

The reason why this is important is that BPA can cause oral and systemic toxicity which has been shown to have estrogenic, cytotoxic, genotoxic, and mutagenic effects on both local tissues and systemically.

BPA belongs to a group of compounds known as xenoestrogens. These compounds have estrogen-mimicking properties and are found in plastics, resins, and methacrylate-based dental materials, including some dental composite resins, dental resin sealants, and bonding agents. Xenoestrogens have been associated with sexual disruption in mammals such as early female puberty, reduced sperm count, and altered function of reproductive organs, as well as increases in breast, ovarian, testicular, and prostate cancer. Other studies have linked xenoestrogen exposure to gestational diabetes, asthma, type 2 diabetes development, altered intestinal permeability, and inflammatory changes in the gut, potentially severe. Pediatric exposure to BPA has been shown to affect reproduction, metabolism, pubertal development, childhood growth, and neurodevelopment. The effects of perinatal and neonatal exposure to estrogenically active compounds have been classified as organizational effects, which can alter existing organs and persist throughout life.

Prenatal exposure to BPA potentially places the fetus at risk for cumulative detrimental effects; the National Toxicology Program and a US Food and Drug Administration risk assessment have stated that "BPA exposure has the potential to alter neurodevelopmental, reproductive, and metabolic end points throughout the lifespan."

There are three routes for systemic absorption of BPA from dental materials: ingestion of released components via the patient's GI tract, diffusion to pulp via dentinal tubules, and uptake of volatile components in the lungs. The long-term leaching of BPA derivatives into the local oral environment and the potential systemic effects are topics of concern. For most individuals, the primary source of exposure to BPA is through diet. Other potential sources include air, dust, water/drinks, and dental restorations. BPA has been found in human blood, urine (2.6 ng/mL), breast milk (1.3 ng/mL), and other tissues. Although the half-life of BPA is reported to be less than 6 hours, some studies suggest that it can be stored in adipose tissue. Although the US Environmental Protection Agency's (EPA) maximum safe dose of BPA is 50 μg/kg body weight/day, animal studies indicate that even low-dose exposure (0.025–2.5 μg/kg body weight/day) could have long-term adverse reproductive, carcinogenic, and other effects.

Studies show that composite restorations (0.25 g) contain less than 500 ng of BPA and will release a small amount of BPA. The BPA concentration in saliva was found to peak over the first several hours after restoration with resin materials but returned to baseline levels within 24–30 hours. The urinary BPA concentration started to increase 9–30 hours after restoration placement. Even if all the BPA is leached out in 1 year, the annual release is still less than the baseline of BPA intake in the United States (from air, dust, water, and food), and is 100 000 ~ 1 000 000 times lower than the EPA maximum safe dose of BPA. The degradation/hydrolysis of Bis-DMA and polycarbonate, however, could lead to a much higher amount of BPA release.

Two factors are involved when considering BPA exposure. The first, as with amalgam restorations, involves the placement and removal of the material. The second, again as with amalgam, involves the leaching of the element/byproduct in question over time.

Composite resins and dental sealants are cured to achieve their final states via free radical chain polymerization with a light catalyst. This conversion of the resin to polymer is technique sensitive. Polymer conversion rates range from 35% for self-curing composites to 77% under laboratory conditions. Even under optimal techniques and conditions, it is reasonable to assume that 23–65% of monomer still remains unpolymerized after curing and thus is freely able to leach into the oral environment. Radical chain polymerization is negatively affected in the presence of oxygen, resulting in an oxygen inhibition layer, where the highest levels of unpolymerized monomer are typically found. There is a direct correlation between the surface area of the restoration and the release of unpolymerized monomer, indicating that large or multiple composite restorations could significantly increase the risk of exposure to BPA derivatives.

Additionally, reduced cure rates secondary to insufficient cure times/intensity significantly increased the solubility and exposure to monomer for many BPA derivative-based resins. For dimethacrylate-based resins, curing times of 80 seconds or more led to greater conversion and less leaching of monomer. Chemically cured formulations, such as those used for core build-ups and restoring areas of the mouth that are difficult for the curing light to reach, have low cure rates, and the possibility of these chemical components leaching out into the oral cavity is increased. Therefore, large composite cores are a cause for concern, as these materials can often remain in the mouth for a long time before they are covered with a definitive restoration. Dual-cure resins obtain a polymerization ratio of only 30–40%. As would be expected, the greatest exposure to uncured resin components occurs immediately after a sealant or composite resin restoration has been placed. It has been suggested that the exposure decreases steadily over time.

The second avenue of exposure is after placement of the restoration. Once composite restorations are placed in the oral environment, they are subject to mechanical wear, as well as enzymatic degradation. The restorations are subject to erosive and abrasive forces through exposure and routine use. These forces will be present for the life of the restoration and put the patient at potential risk for long-term exposure to the resin's components or byproducts.

Cholesterol esterase and pseudocholinesterase will attack the polymer matrix, preferentially hydrolyzing TEGDMA while also hydrolyzing Bis-GMA. Bis-EMA has been used to combat this degradation in some formulations. Other forms of enzymatic attack on the polymer matrix, such as oxidation leading to the release of formaldehyde, could also result in BPA release.In any case, none of these other chemical components have yet been investigated for their potential toxicity in humans. Prenatal exposure to these compounds have the potential to cause life-long effects on immune defenses and predispose female offspring to increased colonic proinflammatory responses such as increased inflammation of the colon, which is also a risk factor for adult development of severe colonic inflammation. *In utero* exposure to estrogenic active chemicals can induce various diseases that might not appear until adulthood. Uterine exposure to endocrine-disrupting chemicals (EDCs), including BPA, predisposes offspring to high birth weight and obesity in adulthood. The *in utero* effect of BPA on cell cycle modification could predispose an individual to a risk of developing diabetes later in life.

The EPA has determined the daily exposure level of BPA of <50 μg/kg (based on toxicity studies involving rodents), although recent rodent studies have shown that levels as low as 10 μg/kg could have detrimental effects such as early-onset puberty, reduced number of offspring, and prostate and urinary changes. A National Toxicology Program (NTP) report concluded that the NTP has "negligible concern that exposure to bisphenol A will cause reproductive effects" and has negligible concern "that exposure of pregnant women to bisphenol A will result in fetal or neonatal mortality, birth defects." The NTP has "some concern for effects on the brain, behavior, and prostate gland in fetuses, infants, and children."

Composite resins containing Bis-DMA or polycarbonate have not been proven to have any adverse human health risks, but more studies should be conducted to evaluate the potential adverse effects of Bis-DMA or polycarbonate-based dental materials. Composite resins containing Bis-GMA or Bis-EMA release BPA far below (0.1%) the daily BPA intake from the environment (dust, air, water) and far below (100 000 ~ 1 000 000 times lower) the EPA maximum safe dose of BPA (50 μg/kg body weight/day), and as such it can safely be stated that they pose no human health risks. On the basis of the benefits of resin-based dental materials and negligible BPA release after resin application, there is no reason to advocate discontinuing their use.

That being said, as with amalgam, it is still prudent to practice the safest means of removing and replacing this material. For as long as the composite resin has been utilized, it has been recommended to remove and place this material using rubber dam isolation. This will give the dentist the ability to protect the resin from moisture, which will affect the cure, and to isolate solvents as well as properly polish the restoration, thereby removing the oxygen inhibition layer. The highest percentage of uncured monomer is present in the oxygen inhibition layer so removing this layer effectively reduces the potential exposure to the patient. To accomplish this, after adjustments have been completed, a cotton pledget placed between a rubber cup and the tooth can be used to remove both the oxygen inhibition layer and the excess amounts of uncured monomer. Rinsing and evacuating/expectorating after the procedure with water for at least 30 seconds will bring leached chemical levels to near baseline.

As in all instances, it is incumbent upon the clinician to learn which product is the safest to use. In the case of composite resin, it is the material that contains acceptable levels of BPA both initially and as the result of degradation. Finally, it is also essential to learn, understand, and implement techniques to minimize exposure.

Treatment of dental disease: take-home message.

- There is no need to obtain the obstetrician's consent in order to perform common dental procedures to a healthy pregnant woman.
- The obstetrician should be informed if a pregnant woman needs to be treated in a hospital setting, especially if the dental procedure requires general anesthesia.
- Be aware of altered bladder habits, aversion to smells and tastes, and increased frequency of exposure to fermentable sugars during pregnancy.
- Manage pregnancy gingivitis through regular dental visits for professional cleaning.
- Periodontal therapy in general and scaling and root planing in particular are safe and appropriate if indicated. Always be aware that gestational diabetes increases the risk of periodontal disease.
- Women should be advised to avoid tooth brushing directly after vomiting as the effect of erosion can be exacerbated by brushing an already demineralized tooth surface.
- Control as many as possible of the conditions that cause or worsen halitosis.
- The degree of periodontal disease and the disturbance of supporting attachment tissues are thought to contribute to tooth mobility during pregnancy, which usually resolves post partum.
- Caries has to be effectively managed to avoid potential complications from tooth decay, with the most important being acute or chronic severe odontalgia and infection. Endodontic treatment in pregnancy should be part of the overall management of dental caries.
- It is generally accepted that it is best to defer elective dental treatment to the second trimester and the first half of the third trimester. Emergency dental procedures are performed without delay and regardless of trimester of pregnancy.
- When a restoration is required during pregnancy, the patient needs to be informed of the different options, so that a consensual decision can be reached on which is the best material to use. Using a rubber dam and high-speed suction during amalgam or composite placement or removal may significantly reduce the inhalation of mercury elements (mercury vapor) and acrylate compounds.

Odontogenic Oral and Maxillofacial Infections in Pregnancy

Kyriaki C. Marti

Pregnancy has been shown to be associated with compromised oral health that can lead to severe odontogenic infections the implications of which in pregnancy can be life-threatening for both the mother and the fetus. The gravid patient is more susceptible to infection for a variety of reasons.

- Potential local causes:
  - Pregnancy gingivitis
  - Periodontitis
  - Periapical lesions due to pulpal necrosis
  - Pericoronitis
- Predisposing factors:
  - Hormonally induced friability of oral mucosa
  - Xerostomia
  - Gestational diabetes
- Corroborating factors:
  - Physiologic changes
  - Other comorbidities

Certain physiologic changes in pregnancy may contribute to the development, severity, and complications of odontogenic infections or to a certain extent facilitate their effective management.

Cardiovascular changes such as increased cardiac output, through the increase in stroke volume as well as the progressive increase in heart rate which peaks in the third trimester, may help to maintain end-organ perfusion until later stages of septic shock. On the other hand, the decrease in blood pressure that usually occurs early in pregnancy (6–8-week gestational age) may decrease the ability of the pregnant patient to compensate for sepsis-related hypotension. As discussed in Chapter 2, the gestational decrease in blood pressure is ascribed to vasodilation mainly caused by relaxin, progesterone, estradiol, and prostacyclin, and potentially by nitric oxide.

Hematologic changes, such as physiologic anemia of pregnancy, may decrease the ability of the pregnant patient to fight infections.

Gastrointestinal changes, particularly gastroesophageal reflux brought about by decreased lower esophageal sphincter pressure, increased abdominal pressure, and slow gastric emptying, increase intraoral acidity with a potential bacterial shift to more acidophilic, cariogenic flora.

Immunologic changes, for reasons discussed in Chapter 2, do not seem to decrease the capacity of the maternal cellular and humoral immunity to combat infections. The majority of papers published on the subject of odontogenic infections in pregnancy refer to maternal immunosuppression as a crucial risk factor. However, the old concept that pregnancy is associated with immune suppression has created a myth of pregnancy as a state of immunological weakness and therefore of increased susceptibility to infectious diseases. Today, there is increasing evidence suggesting that this concept is incorrect and the immune system during pregnancy is functional and highly active (Racicot *et al.* 2014). This concept has been tested for many years in animal models as well as in patients with fertility problems. Unfortunately, after almost 50 years of research following this assumption, there is still lack of evidence to support this hypothesis. Elucidation of the immunologic alterations and adaptations that occur during pregnancy suggests that older concepts of pregnancy as a state of systemic immunosuppression are oversimplified. A more useful model may be the view of pregnancy as a modulated immunologic condition, not a state of immunosuppression. Therefore, it is important to identify (i) whether there is indeed increased susceptibility to infections during pregnancy and (ii) whether there is a difference in the severity of infections.

Although pregnant women are generally not more susceptible to infection, there is solid evidence that if they do become infected, the consequences are more severe. According to Kourtis *et al.* (2014), pregnant women are more severely affected by certain viral infections (influenza, hepatitis E (HEV), herpes simplex virus (HSV)), and malaria parasites compared to nonpregnant women. Evidence is more limited for organisms that cause coccidioidomycosis, measles, smallpox, and varicella (Box 6.4). Furthermore, there are differences in initial susceptibility to infection in pregnant women. Evidence is weaker and is based on reports on the following conditions: malaria (due to *P. falciparum* and *P. vivax*) and listeriosis (*L. monocytogenes*). The authors point out that, regarding malaria, the reported maternal parasitemia, placental parasite burden, and episodes of clinical malaria in areas with a high prevalence of malaria may be associated more with severity than initial susceptibility. Pregnant women have a risk of severe malaria three times higher than that among nonpregnant women. Up to 25% of pregnant women in endemic regions are affected. Increasing parity is associated with decreasing susceptibility to malaria. *Listeria*

Box 6.4 Severity and susceptibility of infections in pregnancy.

Influenza (H1N1) – increased susceptibility in the third trimester

Hepatitis E – high mortality in the third trimester

HSV – increased risk of dissemination and hepatitis

Coccidioidomycosis – incidence decreasing/ pregnant women may not be at increased risk

Measles – increased severity, low susceptibility

Smallpox – increased severity, low susceptibility

Varicella – severity during pregnancy inconclusive

HIV (type 1) – low severity, increased susceptibility

Source: Adapted from Kourtis *et al.* (2014).

has a predilection for the placenta and fetus and, depending on the stage of pregnancy, listeriosis can lead to pregnancy loss, stillbirth, preterm birth, or serious neonatal disease.

Immunologic alterations may help explain this different severity and susceptibility to infectious diseases during pregnancy. These maternal immunologic changes seem to increase the innate immunity of the patient; this may prevent acquisition of infection and explain the absence of increased susceptibility to infections. Still, evidence of increased susceptibility of pregnant women to infection remains weak and relevant controlled studies will be needed in the future.

Odontogenic Oral and Maxillofacial Infections and Their Management

The combination of potential local causes, predisposing, and corroborating factors, as well as the reluctance of health practitioners to treat pregnant women with odontogenic infections, contributes to an exceedingly high risk of these patients developing severe odontogenic infections.

Odontogenic infections can involve primary orofacial and secondary deep neck spaces.

- Primary spaces:
  - Buccal
  - Canine
  - Sublingual
  - Submental
  - Submandibular
  - Vestibular
- Secondary spaces:
  - Infratemporal
  - Lateral pharyngeal
  - Masseteric
  - Masticator
  - Prevertebral
  - Pterygomandibular
  - Retropharyngeal
  - Temporal (superficial and deep)

Severe infections (such as Ludwig's angina) have been reported during pregnancy, with potentially fatal complications when one or more secondary spaces are involved. In particular, the "danger space" (area between the alar and prevertebral fascia extending from the skull base to the diaphragm) and the carotid sheath space (may lead infection to the mediastinum) are anatomic areas of great concern.

Early management of localized mild infections via incision/drainage under local anesthetic with subsequent antibiotic coverage is essential to minimize the risk of infection spreading to the fascial spaces. Exigent, aggressive intervention is the cornerstone of management of severe and deep-space odontogenic infections in pregnancy. An important topic, associated with potentially delayed management of pregnant patients with odontogenic infections, was discussed by Michalowicz *et al.* (2006). According to these authors, dentists may be concerned that bacteremias caused by some dental procedures may lead to uterine infections, spontaneous abortions or preterm labor. Although microorganisms commonly found in the oral cavity have been isolated from amniotic fluid, in cases of chorioamnionitis, "there is no evidence that dental procedure-induced bacteremias increase a woman's risk of experiencing fetal loss or preterm labor and delivery."

Furthermore, potential delay in early management of odontogenic infections may be attributed to the reluctance of some dental practitioners to provide immediate care to pregnant patients. According to Da Costa *et al.* (2010), although many general dentists provide some dental care to pregnant women, more should be done to ensure that this care is comprehensive. It is important to emphasize that the healthy pregnant patient (who is an ASA II category patient, according to the American Society of Anesthesiology) with an uncomplicated pregnancy can be safely treated in an outpatient facility by the general practitioner (within his/her scope of practice and surgical abilities). These patients are often referred for care with written instructions by the OB/GYN specialist or family physician. If no written instructions are available for these patients, the dental practitioner needs to immediately consult the physician, using an effective, secure and legally approved method of communication, after informed consent is given by the patient.

The biggest concern in the management of the pregnant patient is the early recognition of signs and symptoms of metastatic infection that dictate management in a hospital environment (Box 6.5). Severe septic complications that occur in pregnancy are associated with an increased risk of adverse fetal outcomes. Deep-space neck infections (DSNIs) are considered unique among infectious diseases due to their versatility and potential for severe, often life-threatening complications. The complex head and neck anatomy negatively affects early recognition and may delay onset of treatment. Furthermore, a relative increase in cases related to odontogenic infections has been reported, while those caused by pharyngitis or tonsillitis have declined.

Aggressive management of the airway and monitoring are the most urgent and critical aspects of care, followed by appropriate antibiotic coverage and surgical drainage, when needed.

The importance and severity of odontogenic infections, as well as the safety and quality of life of the pregnant patient, require an effective and immediate intervention for treatment, based on the *common principles of therapy*.

- Determine severity of the infection.
- Evaluate host defenses.
- Decide on setting of care.
- Treat surgically.
- Support medically.
- Choose and prescribe antibiotic therapy.
- Administer the antibiotics properly.
- Evaluate the patient frequently.

Box 6.5 Signs and symptoms associated with involvement of secondary spaces.

Fever
Swelling (fluctuant or indurated)
Malaise
Dysphagia
Fatigue
Drooling
Lethargy
Dehydration
Airway compromise
Trismus

Methods commonly used for drainage of an odontogenic infection by the general practitioner are:

- endodontic treatment
- extraction of the offending tooth
- incision and drainage.

Laboratory evaluation includes:

- CBC and differential
- blood cultures (aerobic and anaerobic) should be sent before parenteral antibiotics are given
- needle aspiration of purulent material (for Gram stain, aerobic, anaerobic, and fungal cultures).

Radiographic Examination

Overall, diagnostic radiographic evaluations of the pregnant patient can be safely performed for diagnosis and treatment plan. Still the "lowest amount of reasonably achievable radiation "should be utilized, according to the guidelines published by the ADA in 2012 (Dental Radiographic Examinations: Recommendations for Patient Selection and Limiting Radiation Exposure).

Imaging Methods
- Periapical (PA) radiograph.
- Panoramic radiograph (in a study by Rushton *et al.* (1999), 75.6% of general practitioners were strongly influenced by pregnancy not to take a panoramic radiograph).

Further radiographic evaluation is required when a deep-space infection is present, including:

- ultrasound (US)
- computed tomography (CT) scan
- magnetic resonance imaging (MRI).

Ultrasound examination may offer differential diagnosis between abscess and cellulitis, while digital palpation of the area of concern may reveal the liquid nature of the content and indicate purulent material. A diagnostic ultrasound-guided aspiration may be required for confirmation of diagnosis (Loyer *et al.* 1996).

A CT scan remains the standard of care for diagnosis of deep neck space infections in an emergency setting, and CT scan (with intravenous contrast) is currently the most accurate method to determine location, size, extent, and relationship of the lesion to surrounding structures. The role of emergency CT scan is important in the urgent management of deep-space collections via surgical drainage. However, according to Smith *et al*. (2006), "although CT with contrast plays an important role in the diagnosis and management of DSNIs, the decision for surgical drainage of an abscess should be made clinically."

Magnetic resonance imaging can also be used for the evaluation of DSNIs with a very good degree of accuracy and without the need for contrast medium (see Chapter 4).

Pharmacologic Management of the Patient

Appropriate use of antibiotics and analgesics is essential for a pregnant woman with an odontogenic infection. There is no difference between pregnant and nonpregnant women as to the pharmacologic management of odontogenic infections. As a general rule, the patient should be treated with an empiric antibiotic regimen (taking into consideration any previous history of allergy to antibiotics) until the results of the cultures and sensitivities become available. The reader is referred to Chapter 4 for detailed discussion on antibiotics and analgesics.

Comprehensive Management of Pregnant Patients with Severe Odontogenic Infections

Wong *et al*. (2012) have proposed a useful protocol for the comprehensive management of pregnant patients with severe odontogenic infections. This protocol, with some minor changes (based on our hospital protocol), proposes the following steps.

1) Emergency referral to hospital (when any of the signs and symptoms of a severe infection are present)
2) Medical assessment including maternal airway and fetal health
3) On referral to a tertiary hospital with full specialist teams, consult:
   - Oral and Maxillofacial Surgery (OMS)
   - Obstetrics and Gynecology (O&G)
   - Anesthesia and Intensive Care (A&IC)
4) Admit under the care of the OMS team
5) Control airway (A&IC, OMS – tracheostomy if needed)
6) Full maternal and fetal monitoring (O&G)
7) Infection assessment
8) Airway monitoring
9) Commence intravenous antibiotics (consult: Infectious Diseases – IF)
10) Full specialist assessment by teams
11) Develop plan and gain informed consent:
    - Surgical management
    - Extraction
    - Incision and drainage, cultures (aerobic, anaerobic, fungal, and sensitivities; consult IF with results)
12) Admit to ICU if airway issues (A&IC)
13) Ongoing maternal and fetal monitoring (O&G)
14) General ward until stable
15) Discharge on oral antibiotics
16) Outpatient review by O&G and OMS

Odontogenic oral and maxillofacial infections in pregnancy: take-home message.

- Even the most mild odontogenic infections require early and definitive treatment.
- Any reluctance in treating these infections in pregnancy subjects these patients to an exceedingly high risk of developing severe, life-threatening odontogenic infections.
- Treatment, as long as the conditions allow, should be tailored to maximize the benefit for the mother while minimizing any potential harm to the fetus.
- When faced with odontogenic infections in pregnant women, health practitioners should show no hesitation in referring these patients for timely and appropriate management by a hospital-based multidisciplinary team.

Benign Diseases and Conditions

Christos A. Skouteris

Benign diseases that impact the general population can also affect pregnant women. In addition to dental caries and periodontal disease, benign conditions which require treatment and are pregnancy related include pemphigoid gestationis and the epulis of pregnancy. Certain lesions (e.g., central giant cell granuloma) have been reported as showing an exacerbation during pregnancy, whereas other conditions such as temporomandibular disorders (TMD) show a considerably lower prevalence in pregnant women than nonpregnant women, despite the relationship that TMD and hormones seem to have.

Pregnancy-Related Benign Conditions

Pemphigoid gestationis (PG) is an autoimmune pregnancy-associated subepidermal blistering disease. It usually affects the skin and, rarely, mucous membranes. In the oral cavity, it presents with multiple painful erosions. In rare cases, the oral lesions are prodromal findings before skin lesions develop. Etiologically, the autoimmune response of pregnant patients with predominantly oral mucosal lesions demonstrated the presence of circulating IgA but not IgG autoantibodies, targeting epitopes within the C-terminal portion of the BP180 ectodomain. The lesions of PG cause considerable discomfort during eating and swallowing. Nutritional impairment should be avoided during pregnancy and therefore proper treatment should be instituted. Mild cases can be managed with oral antihistamines or topical corticosteroids. In severe cases with or without generalized skin involvement, treatment consists of administration of steroids (initially prednisolone 50 mg/day), resulting in rapid clearance of both oral and cutaneous lesions that heal without scarring. The corticosteroid dosage is gradually reduced to 25 mg/day to prevent severe exacerbations. The corticosteroids could then be tapered to progressively lower doses and discontinued.

Epulis of pregnancy is a localized, soft, hyperplastic lesion which develops on the gingiva of pregnant women with an estimated incidence of 0.2–5% (Figure 6.1). The epulis is usually pedunculated but can also be broad-based. In its early stages, it is highly vascular with a tendency to bleed spontaneously or when traumatized. The bleeding might be quite excessive not only due to its vascularity but also to a thin overlying epithelium. It may develop at any time during pregnancy but appears to be most common during the second trimester. The lesion usually measures up to 2 cm in diameter but can occasionally grow to a considerable size. Any gingival site can be the location of the epulis but it is mostly found in the interdental papillary labial gingiva of the anterior maxillary teeth. Teeth adjacent to the epulis may become increasingly mobile, although bone around the teeth directly involved by the lesion is very rarely affected.

Histologically, the epulis of pregnancy resembles a pyogenic (telangiectatic) granuloma clinically and histologically. Dental plaque is the spark that can ignite the development of the lesion in addition to hormonal influence. The pregnancy-related hormonal changes that produce an exaggerated gingival

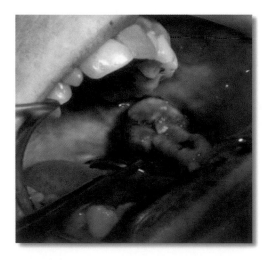

Figure 6.1 Epulis of pregnancy in a patient in her third trimester.

response to plaque are thought to underlie the formation of the pregnancy epulis.

Spontaneous regression of the epulis after birth is common. Surgical removal should only be performed during pregnancy if:

- the epulis is traumatized by opposing teeth or restorations, resulting in pain and bleeding
- it interferes with normal speech and/or mastication
- it becomes painful and bleeds excessively spontaneously without prior trauma.

Surgical removal is also indicated when the epulis does not spontaneously regress in the postpartum period. In addition to surgical removal, contributing local factors should also be addressed. The high recurrence rate of the lesion is mostly due to inadequate management of contributing local factors, such as dental plaque and tartar deposits. Scaling of adjacent teeth should be part of the surgical management of the epulis of pregnancy. Depending on the time of presentation, an asymptomatic epulis of pregnancy can be removed during the second trimester or its removal can be delayed until after delivery, when the epulis may undergo complete spontaneous regression, or might become smaller or more fibrous and therefore easier to remove.

Altered Clinical Behavior of Benign Lesions and Conditions During Pregnancy

Conditions that have been reported to show an increased incidence or an exacerbation during pregnancy include xerostomia, oral candidiasis, geographic tongue (as an oral manifestation of impetigo herpetiformis), and central giant cell granuloma. For the latter, calcitonin appears to be a safe, effective, and conservative treatment for giant cell granulomas that enlarge rapidly during pregnancy.

Studies that have evaluated the evolution of TMD signs and symptoms in women before, during and after pregnancy showed that TMD symptoms previously present decreased during pregnancy and that there was increased mouth opening amplitude during the same period. Reported pain rates, which decreased throughout pregnancy, returned to baseline values in 1 year after delivery. The same was true of estradiol and progesterone levels, an indication of the role of such hormones in modulating pain during pregnancy. Silveira *et al.* (2005) studied the possible association of systemic joint hypermobility and temporomandibular joint (TMJ) hypermobility in pregnant women as a way to establish a higher predisposition to TMD development. Although an association between both conditions was not found, there was a 46% prevalence in TMJ hypermobility during mouth opening among pregnant women.

Cysts and Benign Tumors in Pregnancy

Any type of cyst or benign tumor with or without locally aggressive behavior can potentially occur in pregnancy. Other than sporadic case reports, there are no studies to show that certain cysts or benign tumors show a higher incidence in pregnancy. Case reports on pregnant patients presenting with cystic lesions and benign tumors have included follicular cyst, aneurysmal bone cyst, adenomatoid odontogenic tumor, and ameloblastoma with no evidence-based data on possible hormonal influence.

Surgical treatment during pregnancy poses certain dilemmas, but each case has to be approached on its own merits. Box 6.6 summarizes the author's approach to the management of benign lesions during pregnancy. The approach is not that much different from that of the general population with certain adjustments that the pregnant status mandates. In general, based on the problem at hand and the indicated treatment, procedures may need to be performed irrespective of trimester of pregnancy, delayed until the second trimester, or deferred until post partum.

Box 6.6 Benign diseases and conditions.

Leukoplakia and nonspecific ulcerations – remove possible cause (traumatic or other) and reevaluate in 2 weeks. Biopsy if lesions persist (incisional or excisional based on size, site, and number). If lesion suspicious for malignancy, proceed with biopsy without delay

Cysts of the jaws – acutely infected: treat as an abscess. Defer definitive treatment and follow-up until post partum

Chronically infected with pus-draining fistula (usually from a periapical cyst): endo treatment and follow-up. If lesion persists, extraction of offending tooth or apicoectomy with concomitant enucleation/curettage

Large cystic lesions causing pain, root resorption and mobility of teeth, paresthesia, oral function impairment: aspirate, marsupialize and biopsy. Defer definitive treatment regardless of pathology report (e.g., KOT, mural, luminal ameloblastoma) until post partum and follow up. If malignancy is present or pathologic fracture occurs, treat definitively irrespective of trimester of pregnancy

Soft tissue cysts: mucoceles (if sizeable, traumatized repeatedly, ruptures spontaneously and recurs frequently): unroof and drain content. Ranula: marsupialize. Defer definitive treatment that includes removal of the sublingual gland until post partum

Oral dermoid/epidermoid cysts: if infected treat as an abscess. Defer definitive treatment until post partum unless size and location greatly impair oral function

Branchial cysts/neck dermoids: if infected, treat as an abscess. Defer definitive treatment until post partum unless size and location may cause airway compromise

Benign soft tissue tumors: biopsy (incisional or excisional depending on size). Defer definitive treatment until post partum unless lesion is constantly traumatized, painful, bleeding, and interfering with oral function

Benign locally aggressive solid tumors (e.g., ameloblastoma): based on the usually slow growth rate, surgical treatment can be deferred until post partum under close follow-up throughout pregnancy. However, accelerated growth rate and large lesions that cause malocclusion, displacement of structures (tongue, floor of the mouth, or teeth), are subjected to recurrent trauma due to biting, and with an increased risk of a pathologic fracture require expedient surgical treatment regardless of trimester

Salivary gland disease: acute, recurrent sialadenitis: treat promptly with antibiotics and supportive measures. Defer sialadenectomy (if indicated) until post partum. Sialolithiasis (intraductal or intraparenchymal): asymptomatic – follow-up.Sialolithiasis (intraductal or at the hilum): symptomatic (pain, swelling, and purulent drainage): if stone is not passed and is at the ductal orifice or easily accessible, incise over it and remove. If inaccessible or at the hilum, sialolithectomy via sialoendoscopy

Benign salivary tumors: consider FNAB. Defer definitive treatment until post partum unless the biopsy and certain circumstances dictate otherwise (e.g., sudden size increase, pain, facial nerve weakness)

TMJ/TMD: treat conservatively. Any indicated minimally invasive (arthrocentesis, arthroscopy) or open TMJ procedures are deferred until post partum

Dentofacial abnormalities: orthognathic procedures are deferred until post partum

Cosmetic surgery: cosmetic procedures (invasive or noninvasive) are deferred until post partum

Dentoalveolar surgery: should be performed regardless of trimester only if to extract nonrestorable teeth (with irreversible pulpitis not amenable to endo treatment, causing severe pain and infection), and to repair dentoalveolar traumatic injuries

Important Note: The above described approach to the management of benign lesions during pregnancy is only a reference for the reader's consideration. It does not represent the standard of care in pregnancy, is based on existing surgical principles and clinical judgment, is limited by the relative value of the few existing reports on the subject in the literature, and should be viewed within the context of the surgeon's experience in the treatment of the pregnant patient.

Management of Oral and Maxillofacial Malignancy in Pregnancy

James Murphy and Brent B. Ward

The estimated incidence of cancer diagnosed in pregnant women in developed societies is 1:1000 pregnancies. The most common malignancies affecting pregnant women are:

- ovarian cancer
- cervical cancer
- endometrial cancer*
- vulval cancer*
- pregnancy-associated breast cancer
- Hodgkin lymphoma**
- non-Hodgkin lymphoma
- acute myelogenous leukemia
- acute promyelocytic leukemia
- acute lymphoid leukemia
- melanoma[†]

*Less common, **most common hematologic malignancy in pregnancy, [†]third most common cancer in pregnant women

In the head and neck region, a variety of malignancies have been reported to occur during pregnancy:

- cancer of the larynx
- thyroid cancer
- head and neck melanoma
- head and neck Hodgkin and non-Hodgkin lymphoma
- sinonasal Burkitt lymphoma
- nasopharyngeal carcinoma
- acinic cell carcinoma
- squamous cell carcinoma
- giant cell sarcoma
- ameloblastic carcinosarcoma
- synovial sarcoma
- alveolar rhabdomyosarcoma
- malignant fibrous histiocytoma
- osteosarcoma
- juxtacortical chondrosarcoma.

Head and neck malignancies during pregnancy do not seem to have any association with or any influence from hormonal changes. However, a case report by Al-Zaher and Obeid (2011) documented an acinic cell carcinoma of the parotid which developed in a pregnant woman during her second trimester, treated with superficial parotidectomy. Four years later during the third trimester of a subsequent pregnancy, the patient again developed an acinic cell carcinoma. The authors suggested that this chronologic association might be associated with hormonal and physiologic changes of pregnancy, although chance cannot be ruled out. In support of a hormonal association secondary to pregnancy, estrogen and progesterone receptors have been found in acinic cell carincomas, as reported by Limite *et al.* (2014). Unfortunately, single case reports are unable to answer the relationship of pregnancy with malignancy and large cohort epidemiological studies would be needed.

Oral Cancer in Pregnancy

From the standpoint of the oral health professional, oral cancer in pregnancy, called squamous cell carcinoma (SCCa), is of particular interest. Oral squamous cell carcinoma has been mostly associated with the male gender and older populations. There has been a significant rise in the incidence of tongue squamous cell carcinoma (Box 6.7) among young females, without a history of smoking, and it has been demonstrated that women now tend to delay childbearing to an older age. These two factors have resulted in an increasing prevalence of cancer diagnosed during pregnancy. If the current trends continue, dentists, oral and maxillofacial surgeons as well as obstetricians and gynecologists will see an increasing number of pregnant patients presenting with malignancies.

This in turn leads to a number of complex surgical and adjuvant treatment considerations resulting in ethical and moral decisions for which limited data exist to guide best

Box 6.7 Squamous carcinoma of the tongue – Case in point.

Patient: 29-year-old white female
Gravida: 3
Para: 2
Gestational age at diagnosis: 14 weeks
Biopsy diagnosis: SCCa with perineural invasion
Site: Right tongue, at site of preexisting erythroplakia

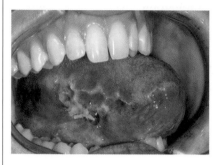

Smoker: No
Alcohol: Occasionally prior to pregnancy
Imaging: MRI – tumor close to midline
–suspicious level 2A lymph node

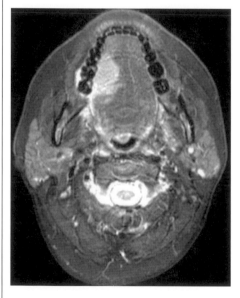

Stage: T4aN1Mx
Consultations: Maternal Fetal Medicine
Tumor Board
Medical Oncology
Radiation Oncology
Nutrition

Treatment plan: Surgery at week 16, chemoradiation
Procedure: Tracheostomy, right hemiglossectomy, bilateral neck dissection, levels I–IV, radial forearm free flap reconstruction
Two teams, duration 471 min, EBL 840 mL
Fetal monitoring: no distress
normal heart tones

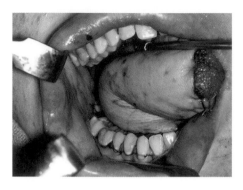

Nutrition: NG feeding tube
Complications: neck wound infection
Management: cepodoxime, clindamycin (2wk)
Final pathology: clear margins, two lymph nodes positive at level IV with extracapsular spread (pT4aN2cMx)
Trach tube, NG tube removed post-op day 18
Radiotherapy with fetal shield, total fetal dose: 7 cGy

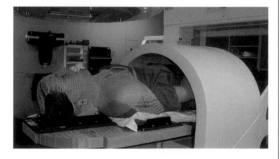

Chemotherapy: Carboplatin (severe nausea, vomiting)
Adjuvant therapy completed at 26 week of gestation
Normal uterine fetal growth on serial ultrasounds
Delivery of a vigorous (3118 g) male infant at 39 weeks
Two-year follow-up: no recurrence
At 2 years the child meets all developmental milestones

practice. The challenge in managing head and neck cancers during pregnancy is the potential counterbalance between maternal and fetal health. Diagnostic and treatment modalities may harm the fetus, while delaying treatment or choosing suboptimal treatment in order to preserve fetal well-being may worsen maternal outcome.

Although the tongue seems to be the predominant location of SCCa during pregnancy, involvement of other sites has also been reported, such as the mucosa of the posterior maxilla, posterior mandible, and the maxillary sinus.

The dichotomy between optimal treatment of the pregnant patient with SCCa and the resultant risks to the fetus represents a complex medical and ethical decision, particularly when long-term impact to the child remains unknown. The patient's decision is a difficult one but has to be respected (see the Angela Carder case in Chapter 1). Multidisciplinary collaboration and communication are key to assist treating providers in their counseling to assure an informed decision. More commonly offered management options include continuation of the pregnancy with standard treatment of the malignancy, continuation of the pregnancy with premature delivery followed by standard treatment, staged approaches (resection of the primary malignancy while pregnant with neck dissection following delivery), as well as termination of pregnancy.

The effect of pregnancy on the malignancy must be considered. Pregnancy induces a number of physiologic changes including immune system modulation, hypercoagulability, hypermetabolism, and decreased albumin with resultant changes in free drug concentrations. Altered hepatic and renal pharmacokinetics additionally have consequences for possible treatments. Conversely, the effect the malignancy has on the pregnancy must also be considered as both conditions place extra nutritional demands on the patient. Additionally, therapies and oncologic interventions have risks

to the pregnancy, including fetal growth restriction, premature delivery, and even intrauterine fetal demise. However, delivery of an unaffected healthy liveborn is possible.

The work-up of the pregnant patient with SCCa should include histopathological confirmation of the diagnosis and radiologic imaging. Pregnancy is not an absolute contraindication to computed tomography of the head and neck with appropriate shielding. MRI in a 1.5 tesla or lower magnetic field without gadolinium would be the preferred imaging modality. Positron emission tomography (PET) used to be considered unsafe in pregnancy. Recent studies have shown, however, that fetal radiation dose from 18 F-FDG PET studies is quite low and significantly below the threshold dose for deterministic effects due to radiation exposure to the fetus. When medically indicated in pregnant patients, 18 F-FDG PET scanning should not be withheld for fear of excessive radiation exposure to the fetus. Dual-modality PET/CT can be safe in pregnancy provided that specific measures are taken to reduce the dose and an analysis of the risk and benefits of the investigation is undertaken.

A multidisciplinary team approach should be adopted in the treatment of these patients. The input of the treating surgeon, radiation oncologist, medical oncologist, maternal fetal medicine physician, speech and language therapist, and nutritionist is essential early in the course of these patients' treatment.

The first case of SCCa of the tongue was reported by Merger and Melchior in 1958. Since that report, 32 more cases, including our own, have been reported in the literature. The demographics of these cases are listed in Box 6.8.

Surgical Considerations

When reviewing published cases, it can be appreciated that surgery has assumed an ever increasing role in the management of these

Box 6.8 Squamous carcinoma of the tongue in pregnancy.

Maternal age: 22–40 (mean: 31 years)
Gestational age at diagnosis: 10–40 weeks (mean 25 weeks)

A) TNM CLASSIFICATION

T	N	M
T1: 6, T2: 15, T3: 3, T4a: 7, T4b: 2	Nx: 1, N0: 17, N1: 4, N2a: 1, N2b: 7, N2c: 2, N3: 1	M not reported: 1, M0: 15, Mx: 17

B) PREGNANCY MANAGEMENT

	Continued	Terminated	Delivery	Cesarean section (C/S)
n:	22*	2**	4	5***

*3 cases ended up with C/S in the 3rd trimester, **one case was a miscarriage, *** C/S performed early or late in 3rd trimester

C) SURGERY

Primary Tumor

	WLE*	Partial glossectomy	Hemiglossectomy	Subtotal glossectomy
n:	8	11	6	1

*WLE: wide local excision

Neck Dissection

	Radical	Modified Radical	Selective
n:	3	1	6 (levels I–III)
			5 (levels I–IV)
			1 (levels I–II)
			3 (levels I–V)

Reconstruction

	RFFF[1]	PTFF[2]	ALTFF[3]	LDFF[4]	RAFF[5]	PMF[6]
n:	5	1	4	1	1	1 (rescue)

[1]Radial forearm free flap, [2]Posterior Tibial, [3]Anterolateral Thigh, [4]Latissimus Dorsi, [5]Rectus Abdominis [6]Pectoralis Major

D) RADIATION (type unspecified): 4, Adjuvant: 7, Brachytherapy: 3
E) CHEMOTHERAPY: 1 (Intra-arterial)
F) CHEMORADIATION: 6

G) TREATMENT OUTCOMES:

	Doing Well	Recurrence (local, regional)	Distant Metastases	Death
Mother n:	22	9	4	10
Child n:	23			

NOTE: Number discrepancies are due to certain data not being stated in some of the reviewed 32 reported cases in the literature patients. The middle trimester of pregnancy is the preferred and likely safest time to perform surgery. The first and third trimesters are less ideal due to the increased risk of miscarriage and deep vein thrombosis respectively. Due to the effects of progesterone on smooth muscle and the increased uterine size, a rapid sequence induction is advisable. Tilting the patient to the left side is advocated during surgery to avoid hemodynamic compromise from inferior vena cava compression. Surgery should be performed in an expedited fashion with care taken to minimize blood loss.

Defect Reconstruction

The defects resulting from tumor resection in pregnant women have been reconstructed with split-thickness skin grafts, regional, and free tissue transfers. Temporalis and pectoralis major flaps have been used successfully for this purpose as regional flaps. Free tissue transfers have included the radial forearm, anterolateral thigh, posterior tibial, latissimus dorsi, rectus abdominis, and free fibula osteocutaneous flaps. Successful microvascular tissue transfer involves a two-team approach and a high level of technical expertise with close cooperation between surgical and anesthesia teams. The two-team approach reduces the operating time and hence prolonged exposure of mother and fetus to the anesthetics and surgical stress.

A potential surgical difficulty related particularly to free tissue transfers is the hypercoaguable state of pregnancy that increases the risk of thromboembolic disease and anastomotic thrombosis. Pregnancy increases the concentration of clotting factors, including I (fibrinogen), II (prothrombin), VII (proconvertin), VIII (antihemophilic factor A), IX (Christmas factor), X (plasma thromboplastin antecedent), XI (plasma thromboplastin antecedent), plasminogen, and D-dimer, speeds turnover of platelets,

and reduces fibrinolytic activity, all of which contribute to thrombosis. This can be successfully prevented with the prophylactic use of low molecular weight heparin, which does not cross the placenta or have teratogenic effects.

Regarding the physiologic hemodynamic changes occurring in pregnancy, the increase in cardiac output and stroke volume and the decrease in peripheral vascular resistance do not seem to increase blood loss during surgery and may help to maintain anastomotic patency.

Fetal Monitoring

Intraoperative continuous electronic fetal monitoring (FM) may be considered during nonobstetric procedures of long duration and when intervention on behalf of a viable fetus would ensue if intraoperative fetal compromise was noted. There are two types of electronic fetal monitoring: external and internal. Standard external electronic fetal monitors have two main components applied with belts over the abdomen: a Doppler ultrasound transducer that monitors the fetal heart rate (fetal cardiotocograph) and a tocodynamometer used to assess for uterine contractions. These are connected with a cable to a central unit that provides tracings as well as audible and visual signals. Wireless fetal monitors that utilize conductive patches and electrodes as well as Bluetooth connectivity are also available. Internal fetal monitoring is only implemented when the amniotic sac is ruptured, the cervix is dilated, and delivery is in progress. The ACOG fetal monitoring guidelines are discussed in Chapter 4.

Radiotherapy

Radiotherapy can be used as primary treatment or in the adjuvant setting for SCCa of the tongue in pregnant patients due to the distance of the target site from the fetus. The radiation dose to which the fetus is exposed results from the relative contribution of radiation leakage and scatter radiation, including head scatter and internal scatter. The use of abdominal shields can reduce radiation leakage and scatter significantly.

Volumetric modulated arc therapy (VMAT) was used in our patient to reduce the dose to the fetus. In comparison to intensity modulated radiotherapy (IMRT) treatment that resulted in a similar dose distribution, the VMAT plan resulted in fewer monitor units, thereby reducing the effects of radiation leakage and resultant dose to the fetus, without compromising therapy to the targeted site. A further benefit of VMAT compared to IMRT was the comparatively shorter time required to deliver an equivalent dose of radiation which minimizes the length of time the pregnant patient has to lie flat. As the fetus is exposed to increasing radiation doses, higher potential short- and long-term complications exist. The fetus is most vulnerable to the effects of radiation during organogenesis in the first trimester. Guidelines from the American Association of Physicists in Medicine state the risk to the fetus is not significant below a dose of 5 cGy and unlikely to be significant below a dose of 10 cGy. There is no observable effect on fetal development as assessed by developmental delay, gross malformations, or growth restriction, which could be separated from the underlying spontaneous rate, when a fetus is exposed to such low doses. The dose of 7 cGy in the presented case is unlikely to have any significant effects on the fetus. The stochastic effect of radiation must be acknowledged with an estimate of the relative risk of childhood cancer and leukemia at 1.4 per cGy.

Chemotherapy

Administration of chemotherapy during pregnancy exposes the fetus to greatest risk during the first trimester. Concerns about the administration of cytotoxic chemotherapy during pregnancy arise because chemotherapy preferentially kills rapidly proliferating cells like the fetal mass. This is especially true during the first 8 weeks post conception. After organogenesis, the genitalia, central nervous system, and hematopoietic system remain vulnerable to continued exposure but the use of chemotherapy in the second and third trimesters has been demonstrated to be safe.

Platinum derivatives do cross the placenta where they can result in potential teratogenicity. Cisplatin is frequently used in the adjuvant treatment of oral cavity SCCa when National Comprehensive Cancer Network (NCCN) guidelines are met. Mhallem Gziri *et al.* (2013) reported on the use of adjuvant chemoradiation with cisplatin in a patient with tongue SCCa during pregnancy without complication. The patient reported in the current case received carboplatin due to its reported better toxicity profile compared to cisplatin in the context of pregnancy. Doses of carboplatin up to an area under the curve of 7.5 have been shown not to be associated with significant placental transfer, fetal exposure or fetal toxic effects in an *ex vivo* study. Increased risk of intrauterine growth restriction and low birth weight has been associated with exposure to these agents during pregnancy. As platinum agents cross the placenta, delivery should be delayed for 3 weeks after the last dose to allow fetal drug excretion as well as subsequent rise in the fetal hematologic counts and profile.

No cases of secondary leukemia have been reported in the literature in those who were exposed to chemotherapy *in utero*. However, extrapolating data from children, it would seem logical that there would be an increased risk of leukemia and lymphoma.

In summary, patients with oral malignancy may undergo standard of care treatment with appropriate consent and modifications which protect both the mother and fetus. Careful collaboration of a team of surgical and medical oncologists as well as maternal fetal medicine specialists is optimal for patient management in this complex situation.

Management of oral and maxillofacial malignancy in pregnancy: take-home message.

The estimated incidence of cancer diagnosed in pregnant women in developed societies is 1:1000 pregnancies.

The most common malignancies affecting pregnant women are ovarian and cervical cancer, pregnancy-associated breast cancer, lymphoma, leukemia, and melanoma.

Head and neck malignancies during pregnancy do not seem to have any association with or any influence from hormonal changes.

There has been a significant rise in the incidence of tongue squamous cell carcinoma among young females, without a history of smoking.

The tongue seems to be the predominant location of SCCa during pregnancy.

The dichotomy between optimal treatment of the pregnant patient with SCCa and the resultant risks to the fetus represents a complex medical and ethical decision. The patient's decision is a difficult one but has to be respected.

Therapies and oncologic interventions have risks to the pregnancy, including altered fetal growth with resultant fetal growth restriction, premature delivery, and even intrauterine fetal demise. However, delivery of an unaffected healthy liveborn is possible.

Magnetic resonance imaging in a 1.5 tesla or lower magnetic field without gadolinium would be the preferred imaging modality.

18F-FDG PET scanning should not be withheld for fear of excessive radiation exposure to the fetus and dual-modality PET/CT can be safe for use in pregnancy.

The input of the treating surgeon, radiation oncologist, medical oncologist, maternal fetal medicine physician, speech and language therapist, and nutritionist is essential early in the course of treatment.

Tilting the patient to the left side is advocated during surgery to avoid hemodynamic compromise from inferior vena cava compression. Surgery should be performed in an expedited fashion with care taken to minimize blood loss.

A potential surgical difficulty related particularly to free tissue transfers is the hypercoagulable state of pregnancy that increases the risk of thromboembolic disease and anastomotic thrombosis.

Intraoperative continuous electronic fetal monitoring may be considered during nonobstetric procedures of long duration.

American Association of Physicists in Medicine guidelines state that the risk to the fetus during radiotherapy is not significant below a dose of 5 cGy and unlikely to be significant below a dose of 10 cGy.

Carboplatin seems to have a better toxicity profile compared to cisplatin in the context of pregnancy. Doses of carboplatin up to an area under the curve of 7.5 have been shown not to be associated with significant placental transfer, fetal exposure or fetal toxic effects.

Management of Oral and Maxillofacial Trauma in Pregnancy

Igor Makovey and Sean P. Edwards

Epidemiology

Trauma is the leading cause of nonobstetric maternal death, with placental abruption being the most common contributing factor. Fildes *et al.* (1992) stated that 50% of maternal deaths are due to trauma, 6–7% of all pregnancies are complicated by trauma, and 0.4% of pregnant patients require hospitalization in order to treat traumatic injuries. In general, the various causes for trauma that result in injury and death during pregnancy are not that much different from the general population. Motor vehicle accidents account for more than 50% of all cases of trauma during pregnancy and 82% of traumatic fetal deaths. Other reported causes of maternal injury include:

- assault
- gunshots
- stabbing
- strangulation
- falls
- suicide
- drug overdose
- poisoning
- burns.

Major blunt and penetrating trauma are more likely to affect both a pregnant woman and her fetus.

Pregnancy-specific injuries, such as placental abruption and fetal injuries, can occur after relatively minor trauma to the abdomen from falls, domestic abuse, and even low-speed motor vehicle accidents. Violence deserves special attention since the incidence seems to increase during pregnancy. Stewart and Cecutti (1993) reported an incidence of 6.6% physical abuse in pregnancy, which is markedly elevated compared to general population rates. Other studies have reported significantly higher frequencies of abuse at 10–30%, with 5% of those resulting in fetal death. The predispos-

ing factors of intimate partner violence were noted to be patients younger than 25 years of age, less educated patients, and lower socioeconomic class. The oral and maxillofacial surgeon is often the first practitioner to see and evaluate these patients and should be prepared to identify and appropriately refer victims of domestic violence to prevent future injuries. It is our obligation as healthcare providers to question each injured women about intimate partner violence and safety at home in the absence of the intimate or domestic partner.

Injuries to the head and neck are common, with an annual incidence approaching 5 million in the United States. There is no reported incidence of head and neck injuries in pregnant women though underreporting is likely since not all pregnant patients will present to a physician with an injury and not all patients with an injury to the head and neck will have a pregnancy test. To optimize the management of the pregnant patient with a neck injury, it is imperative to understand the risks and benefits associated with management of the pregnant patient. The Advanced Trauma Life Support (ATLS) protocols remain the standard of care in the pregnant patient.

Primary Survey

According to ATLS guidelines, best treatment for the fetus is optimal resuscitation of the mother. However, clinicians treating injured pregnant patients are obligated to be aware of the fetus and the influence it has on maternal physiology. Provision of optimal care in a pregnant patient commands a multidisciplinary team approach involving emergency medicine physicians, trauma surgeons, obstetricians, and neonatologists. The primary survey is typically executed by emergency physicians and includes establishment of patent airway, adequate ventilation, and circulation.

Gravid patients are at an increased risk for airway complications and are noted to be eight times more likely to have a failed intubation. Several anatomic and physiologic changes that accompany pregnancy are responsible for this difficulty. Weight gain during pregnancy is common and a well-known risk factor for difficult intubation. Increased maternal progesterone has been implicated in development of friable and edematous oral and pharyngeal mucosa. Friable edematous mucosa is prone to bleeding during intubation, which may further compromise the clinician's ability to secure the airway. Further complicating intubation is the increased risk of gastroesophageal reflux and aspiration in the gravid patient. The increased maternal progesterones and decreased motilin reduce lower esophageal sphincter tone and, in some, delay gastric emptying. Further exacerbating the situation is the increased intraabdominal pressure from the gravid uterus. Given the changes and the fact that trauma itself delays gastric emptying, securing the airway of an injured pregnant patient mandates a rapid sequence intubation. Additionally, increased gastric acid content in the oropharynx due to the decreased lower esophageal sphincter tone contributes to an increased risk of aspiration before and during the intubation.

There is a 30–40% increase in minute ventilation in the setting of increased tidal volumes with an unchanged respiratory rate in a gravid patient. This is mostly attributed to a 20–30% increase in oxygen consumption and CO_2 production during pregnancy. Furthermore, circulating progesterone directly stimulates the central respiratory center and leads to mild respiratory alkalosis. Although there is a rise in carbon dioxide production, the tremendous increase in minute ventilation leads to a decrease in partial pressure of carbon dioxide in arterial blood. Normal values are 30–35 mmHg ($PaCO_2$ 30–35). Thus, a pregnant patient with carbon dioxide partial pressure of 40 mmHg ($PaCO_2$ 40) may be a strong candidate for invasive or noninvasive mechanical ventilation in order to improve minute ventilation and carbon dioxide clearance.

Blood volume is increased by 40% or up to 2 L during pregnancy. This tremendous increase contributes to a delay in clinical manifestation of hemodynamic instability while in a state of hypovolemia. This increase in volume leads to a dilutional anemia which is also accompanied by a decrease in colloid oncotic pressure so that the pregnant patient is also more susceptible to heart failure.

As mentioned previously, placental abruption is the most common cause of maternal death in a trauma setting. This can be thought of as a hemorrhagic condition between the placenta and uterus, leading to compromise of placental perfusion. Placental abruption is suspected clinically when a pregnant patient presents with a triad of sudden onset of antepartum vaginal bleeding, severe tenderness of the uterus, and hypertonic uterine contractions. However, maternal vital signs may be preserved at the expense of placental perfusion. In the setting of increased blood volume, the mother may lose up to 1.5 L of blood prior to manifestation of tachycardia and hypotension as signs of hypovolemic shock. Notably, fetal distress may be the first sign of maternal hypovolemia.

Thus fetal heart tone monitoring with an ultrasound Doppler and uterine contraction monitoring with a tocodynamometer should be initiated as soon as possible in the traumatized gravid patient. The acceptable fetal heart rate range is 120–160 beats per minute. Fetal signs of distress include an abnormal heart rate, heart rate decelerations or absence of accelerations, and frequent uterine contractions. These manifestations may represent fetal hypoxia and acidosis and may require prompt interventions. If maternal and fetal vital signs continue to deteriorate with adequate resuscitation, an emergent cesarean delivery may be indicated. When evaluating maternal vital signs, clinicians should always be aware of uterine compression of the inferior vena cava from the gravid uterus when a pregnant patient is left supine, reducing blood return to the right side of the heart by 30% and exacerbating or mimicking hypovolemic states.

Preterm Labor

Preterm labor may be a direct result of traumatic injury or may manifest as a result of placental abruption. Irrespective of cause, there is a two-fold increase in preterm delivery in injured patients. Preterm labor can be diagnosed with a tocodynamometer and clinical examination. It should be considered when regular and frequent contractions are noted.

If preterm labor is suspected, speculum examination must be performed and cervical dilation determined. Cervical dilation of more than 3 cm and effacement (stretching and thinning of the cervix) of more than 80% support manifestation of preterm labor. In women less than 34 weeks of gestation, treatment of preterm labor is initiated, the goal of which is to delay delivery in order to assist with pulmonary fetal development. Magnesium sulfate is used to promote tocolysis (postponement of preterm labor). Systemic steroids are used to encourage neonatal pulmonary development and reduce morbidity and mortality. Women who are more than 34 weeks of gestation do not require inhibition of acute preterm labor and are typically allowed to proceed with delivery.

Alloimmunization

Even with minor injury, all Rh-negative pregnant patients are at risk of Rh alloimmunization. The incidence of maternal fetal hemorrhage has been noted to be 10–30% in all injured women. The vast majority of maternal fetal hemorrhages are subclinical and may lead to future development of Rh disease of the newborn. In order to prevent this complication, anti-D IgG should be given to all Rh-negative pregnant women within 72 hours of injury. A single dose protects against sensitization for up to 30 mL of fetal blood, which is sufficient in 90% of maternal-fetal hemorrhages. Further, the Kleihauer–Betke (KB) test may be performed to evaluate for hemorrhage in excess of 30 ml and the need for an additional dose of Anti-D IgG. Kleihauer–Betke testing, which measures the amount of fetal hemoglobin transferred from a fetus to a mother's bloodstream, accurately predicts the risk of preterm labor after maternal trauma. Clinical assessment does not. With a negative KB test, posttrauma electronic fetal monitoring duration may safely be limited. With a positive KB test, the significant risk of preterm labor mandates detailed monitoring. KB testing has important advantages for all maternal trauma victims, regardless of Rh status.

Ionizing Radiation

It is important to confirm with an obstetrician the risks and benefits of radiologic interventions. However, if one is not available, indicated radiographic studies should be performed. Clinicians commonly hesitate when ordering imaging studies for pregnant patients due to concern about teratogenicity, restriction of fetal growth, and CNS development. However, radiation exposures from the imaging used for an injured pregnant patient have a very low risk to the developing fetus, especially when performed in the head and neck area. It should be common practice to protect the uterus from ionizing radiation with a lead apron when possible (see Chapter 4).

Secondary Survey (Oral Cavity, Maxillofacial Region, and Neck)

An oral and maxillofacial surgeon may have a role in the primary survey which includes establishment of the airway and control of hemorrhage. This may involve intubation, emergent cricothyrotomy or tracheostomy, and achieving control of hemorrhage. Once the airway, ventilation, and circulation have been established, the secondary survey proceeds with sequential examination of the head, neck, maxillofacial region, and oral cavity.

During head evaluation, the entire scalp should be examined for lacerations, hemorrhages, and bony deformities. The scalp is a highly vascular site and a common area of significant blood loss. Ears must be examined for lacerations, exposure of cartilage, and loss of hearing. Otoscopic examination of the external auditory canal and tympanic membrane should be accomplished as well. Bruising and lacerations should be noted as they may indicate a fracture. Hemotympanum can be an early sign of basal skull fracture. The Battle sign, known to be an indicator of basilar skull fracture, is defined as retroauricular ecchymosis which appears 1–3 days after sustaining fracture. Similarly, periorbital ecchymosis, classically known as "raccoon eyes," indicative of an interior cranial base fracture, is typically not present on examination immediately following the injury but appears 1–3 days after injury. Other signs of basilar skull fracture include clear rhinorrhea or otorrhea indicating cerebrospinal fluid (CSF) leakage. Patients may report a salty taste in their mouth in association with CSF rhinorrhea.

Early ophthalmic examination is indicated before edema sets in. This should include evaluation of visual acuity, pupillary size, conjunctival hemorrhages, fundi and assessment of dislocation of the ocular axial length (indicative of intraocular lens dislocation). If a patient presents with eye pain, pressure, changes in vision, new-onset proptosis, and relative afferent pupillary defect, the clinician must suspect retrobulbar hematoma. This is a clinical diagnosis and when suspected, the patient should undergo ocular tonometry to assess ocular pressures. If ocular pressure is elevated above 30 mmHg, emergent lateral canthotomy and inferior cantholysis must be performed. Diplopia in superior gaze and inability to move the eye cranially after facial trauma likely represent entrapment of inferior rectus, suggestive of orbital floor fracture. This is an indication for immediate surgical intervention if the patient is systemically stable.

Prior to performing an intraoral examination, it is helpful to appreciate any swelling, asymmetry, lacerations, or ecchymosis of the lips. This may provide the first clue to concomitant dentoalveolar trauma. Initially, a generalized evaluation of the integrity of the oral mucosa and dentition should be performed, looking for avulsed/ fractured dentition, expanding hematoma, tongue elevation, or uvula deviation that may compromise the airway. Transorally, the maxilla and mandible should be palpated in order to evaluate for bony discontinuity and step-offs. It is prudent to palpate the floor of the mouth as alveolar and, more commonly, mandibular fractures can present with a sublingual hematoma. The mobility of the maxilla should be evaluated by placing one hand pinched over the bridge of the nose for traction and the other hand grasping the premaxilla. Mobility of the maxilla would suggest a LeFort fracture and would warrant further imaging. An examination of the dentition should include the position of each tooth as it relates to the arch form both anterior/posterior and incision/apically. Depending on the vector of the traumatic force, the dentition may be subluxated, intruded or avulsed. The ability to mobilize a segment of multiple teeth separate from the remaining dentition is highly indicative of an alveolar fracture. Knowing whether a tooth or multiple teeth are subluxated or part of an alveolar fracture would change the rigidity of the splinting and duration needed. Pulp testing is typically delayed for subsequent follow-up appointments as false negatives are common immediately following trauma and would add little to the initial management.

Maxillofacial bones should be palpated thoroughly, but if not involved with airway obstruction, definitive management may be safely delayed until after the patient is stabilized and life-threatening injuries are addressed. When evaluating nasal structures, it is important to perform a speculum examination and assess for septal hematoma. This should be treated emergently with a small incision to drain the blood in order to prevent future septal perforation and saddle nose deformity.

The neck should be inspected for signs of blunt and penetrating injury, tracheal deviation, and use of accessory respiratory muscles. Next, palpation is performed to assess for tenderness, deformity, swelling, subcutaneous emphysema, tracheal deviation, and symmetry of pulses. The carotid arteries are auscultated for bruits. A CT scan of the cervical spine or a lateral, cross-table cervical spine X-ray should be obtained and adequate in-line immobilization and protection of the cervical spine should be maintained until the cervical spine is cleared for injuries.

Oral and Maxillofacial Surgical Considerations (Box 6.9)

Essentially, there is no difference in the way maxillofacial trauma is managed in pregnancy compared with the way these injuries are treated in the general population, provided that certain steps precede the decision

Box 6.9 Oral and maxillofacial trauma – Case in point.

Patient: 17-year-old female
Gravida: 1
Para: 0
Gestational age: 29 weeks
Cause of injuries: MVA
Contributing factors: Unrestrained passenger
Ejected through windshield
Condition on-scene: ambulating, agitated,
combative

Transfer to first-line hospital
Condition: Altered mental status
Airway compromise
Management: Intubation
Imaging: CT scan (head, maxillofacial region,
c-spine, thoracic spine, chest X-ray
Findings: no intracranial hemorrhage,
no bony structural abnormalities
c-spine, thoracic spine, and chest X-ray
OB-GYN findings: cervix dilated 2 cm,
contraction q 4–5 min
no vaginal bleeding
Patient given 1 dose of betamethasone in
preparation for preterm labor

Transfer to CS Mott Children's Hospital
En route: hypotensive, bradycardic
received 3% saline solution

At CS Mott Children's Hospital ED
Vital signs: BP: 150/99, HR: 24, SpO$_2$: 99% on
100% FiO$_2$
Primary survey: extensive facial soft tissue trauma

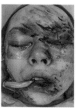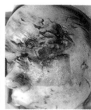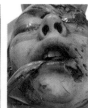

Secondary survey:
Large skin avulsion, left supraorbital rim,
avulsion lateral to the left commissure,
numerous forehead and cheek lacerations,
complete function of CN VII,
bilateral epistaxis consistent with CT scan finding
of minimally displaced nasal bone fracture,
bilateral medial wall maxillary sinus fractures.

At CS Mott Children's Hospital ED
Neurologic exam: noncontributory – patient
sedated
OB-GYN sterile vaginal exam: contractions
q 1–2 min
Fetal heart sounds 130, occasionally
variable
Repeat CT scan: no findings other than the
nasal injury

Admission to Pediatric Surgical ICU
OB-GYN: Serial SVE and fetal monitoring
Obstetric clearance for surgical repair of
facial injuries
Obstetricians, neonatology standing by

Operating Room
Surgical repair in progress
Fetal monitoring: bradycardia, HR: 90/min
SEV: progression of labor, birth center called
Emergent low transverse C-section
performed
Infant APGAR score: 0 on presentation
1 at 1 min, 1 at 5 min
Umbilical cord pulse: not palpable
Infant CPR initiated, intubation, epinephrine,
HR: >100/min
Infant NICU admission
Postop maternal condition: good
Infant condition: Treatment for respiratory
distress
Mother discharged, infant discharged 1
month later
5-month follow-up:

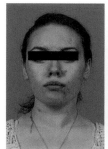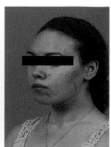

Patient is to undergo scar revision in the near
future

to intervene. Maternal and fetal stability has to be ascertained and obstetric consultation and clearance will be required in all pregnant trauma patients. Obstetric involvement would also determine the need for continuous electronic fetal monitoring. The patient's airway has to be protected and secured. There should be no hesitation in intubating the patient or providing a surgical airway (tracheotomy) when there is indication that the patient's breathing is or could be compromised. Once the spine is cleared from injury, the gravid trauma patient should be kept in the left lateral decubitus position to avoid aortocaval compression and supine hypotensive syndrome.

Even if a pregnant patient presents to the dental office with only avulsed teeth with or without associated dentoalveolar fracture, secondary to a fall or domestic violence, she should be referred to the hospital for evaluation and treatment. Since it is prudent to assume that force could also have been applied to the abdomen, hospital referral is justified because complications limited to the pregnancy itself, such as an abruption, can occur after even relatively minor trauma to the abdomen from falls, domestic abuse, and low-speed motor vehicle accidents.

If facial fractures are present, rigid fixation of maxillary and mandibular fractures is advisable to avoid or minimize the period of maxillomandibular fixation (MMF). This approach allows the restoration of adequate nutrition as rapidly as possible and minimizes aspiration risk. If maxillomandibular fixation is necessary, the newly introduced hybrid MMF systems or MMF screws should be used and elastic bands applied. The use of elastic bands provides a quick release from fixation in case of nausea and vomiting. In addition, the patient can be instructed to remove and replace them, if fracture stability allows and oral intake is not contraindicated. Otherwise, parenteral nutrition supplementation should be considered.

Finally, as another option, fracture treatment could be temporized with closed reduction until post partum, at which time definitive treatment could be performed, particularly if the patient's gestation is nearing completion.

Management of oral and maxillofacial trauma in pregnancy: take-home message.

Trauma continues to be the leading cause for non-obstetric maternal death, with placental abruption being the most common contributing factor.

Motor vehicle accidents account for more than 50% of all cases of trauma during pregnancy and are responsible for 82% of fetal deaths caused by trauma.

Gravid patients are at an increased risk for airway complications and are noted to be eight times more likely to have a failed intubation.

In the trauma setting, electronic fetal monitoring should be initiated as soon as possible.

Irrespective of cause, there is a two-fold increase in preterm delivery in injured patients.

Even with minor injury, all Rh-negative pregnant patients are at risk of Rh alloimmunization.

Radiation exposures from imaging used for an injured pregnant patient have a very low risk to the developing fetus, especially when performed in the head and neck area with proper shielding.

Intraoral exam has to be performed carefully because the oral and oropharyngeal mucosa is more friable and hemorrhagic than normal as a result of gestational hormonal changes.

There is no difference in the way maxillofacial trauma is managed in pregnancy compared with the way these injuries are treated in the general population, provided that certain steps precede the decision to intervene.

Complications limited to pregnancy itself, such as abruption placenta and fetal injuries, can occur after even relatively minor trauma to the abdomen from falls, domestic abuse, and low-speed motor vehicle accidents.

Rigid fixation of maxillary and mandibular fractures is advisable to avoid or minimize the period of maxillomandibular fixation.

If maxillomandibular fixation is necessary, the newly introduced hybrid MMF systems or MMF screws should be used and elastic bands applied.

References

Al-Zaher NN and Obeid AA. (2011) Acinic cell carcinoma in pregnancy: a case report and review of the literature. *Journal of Medical Case Reports*, **5**, 91.

Da Costa EP, Lee JY, Rozier RG, *et al.* (2010) Dental care for pregnant women. *Journal of the American Dental Association*, **141**, 986.

Fildes J, Reed L, Jones N, *et al.* (1992) Trauma: the leading cause of nonobstetric maternal death. *Journal of Trauma*, **32**, 643.

Kourtis AP, Read JS, and Jameson DJ. (2014) Pregnancy and infection. *New England Journal of Medicine*, **370**, 2211–2218.

Limite G, di Micco R, Esposito E, *et al.* (2014) Acinic cell carcinoma of the breast: review of the literature. *International Journal of Surgery*, **12**, S35.

Loyer EM, DuBrow RA, David CL, *et al.* (1996) Imaging of superficial soft-tissue infections: sonographic findings in cases of cellulitis and abscess. *American Journal of Roentgenology*, **166**, 149.

Merger R and Melchior J. (1958) Pregnancy occurring in a woman with cancer of the tongue: ulceration of the internal carotid artery. *Bulletin de la Federation des Societes de Gynecologie et d'Obstetrique de Langue Francais*, **10**, 270.

Michalowicz BS, Hodges JS, DiAngelis AJ, *et al.* (2006) Treatment of periodontal

disease and the risk of preterm birth. *New England Journal of Medicine*, **355**, 1885.

Mhallem Gziri M, Han SN, van Calsteren K, *et al.* (2013) Tongue cancers during pregnancy: case reports and review of literature. *Head and Neck*, **35**, E102.

Racicot K, Kwon JY, Aldo P, *et al.* (2014) Understanding the complexity of the immune system during pregnancy. *American Journal of Reproductive Immunology*, **72**, 107.

Rushton VE, Horner K, and Worthington HV. (1999) Factors influencing the selection of panoramic radiography in general dental practice. *Journal of Dentistry*, **27**, 565.

Silveira EB, Rocabado M, Russo AK, *et al.* (2005) Incidence of systemic joint hypermobility and temporomandibular joint hypermobility in pregnancy. *Cranio*, **23**, 138.

Smith J L, Hsu JM, and Chang J. (2006) Predicting deep neck space abscess using computed tomography. *American Journal of Otolaryngology*, **27**, 244.

Stewart DE and Cecutti A. (1993) Physical abuse in pregnancy. *Canadian Medical Association Journal*, **149**, 1257.

Wong D, Cheng A, Kunchur R, *et al.* (2012) Management of severe odontogenic infections in pregnancy. *Australian Dental Journal*, **57**, 498.

Further Reading

Abramowicz S, Abramowicz JS, and Dolwick MF. (2006) Severe life threatening maxillofacial infection in pregnancy presented as Ludwig's angina. *Infectious Diseases in Obstetrics and Gynecology*, Article ID 51931, 1–4.

Achtari MD, Georgakopoulou EA, and Afentoulide N. (2012) Dental care throughout pregnancy. What a dentist must know. *Oral Health and Dental Management*, **11**, 169.

Acquah L and Burton R. (2014) Obstetric medicine. Interlinking obstetrics and

internal medicine. *South African Medical Journal*, **104**, 636.

Adetayo AM, Oyedele TA, Sodipo BO, *et al.* (2017) Management of severe orofacial infections. Report of two cases and literature review. *International Journal of Infectious and Tropical Diseases*, **4**, 18.

Afzalinasab S, Mahdieh Taleb M, Khajehahmadiet S, *et al.* (2015) Maxillary sinus squamous cell carcinoma during pregnancy. a new case report. *Cumhuriyet Dental Journal*, **18**, 364.

Amant F, van Calsteren K, Halaska MJ, *et al.* (2009) Gynecologic cancers in pregnancy. Guidelines of an International Consensus Meeting. *International Journal of Gynecological Cancer*, **19**, S1.

American College of Surgeons (2013) *Advanced Trauma Life Support (ATLS). Student* Manual, 9th edn, American College of Surgeons, Washington DC, p. 25.

ASA Physical Status Classification System. Available online at: www.asahq.org/ resources/clinical-information/asa-physical-status-classification-system (accessed 20 October 2017).

Ask K, Akesson A, Berglund M, *et al.* (2002) Inorganic mercury and methylmercury in placentas of Swedish women. *Environmental Health Perspectives*, **110**, 523.

Atabo A and Bradley PJ. (2008) Management principles of head and neck cancers during pregnancy. A review and case series. *Oral Oncology*, **44**, 236.

Atkinson LA, Santolaya J, Matta P, *et al.* (2015) The sensitivity of the Kleihauer–Betke test for placental abruption. *Journal of Obstetrics and Gynecology*, **35**, 139.

Bansal S, Kumar L, Choudhary N, *et al.* (2015) Osteosarcoma of mandible in pregnancy – a management challenge. *Online Journal of Health and Allied Sciences*, **14**, 6. Available online at: www.ojhas.org/issue53/2015-1-6.html (accessed 20 October 2017).

Basavaraju A, Vijaya Durga S, and Vanitha B. (2012) Variations in the oral anaerobic microbial flora in relation to pregnancy. *Journal of Clinical and Diagnostic Research*, **6**, 1489.

Bearfield C, Davenport ES, Sivapathasundaram V, *et al.* (2002) Possible association between amniotic fluid micro-organism infection and microflora in the mouth. *British Journal of Obstetrics and Gynaecology*, **109**, 527.

Bhandari N and Kothari M. (2010) Adenomatoid odontogenic tumour mimicking a periapical cyst in pregnant woman. *Singapore Dental Journal*, **31**, 26.

Boatin AA, Wylie B, Goldfarb I, *et al.* (2015) Wireless fetal heart rate monitoring in inpatient full-term pregnant women. Testing functionality and acceptability. *PLoS One*, **10**, e0117043, 2015.

Bradley PJ and Raghavan U. (2004) Cancers presenting in the head and neck during pregnancy. *Current Opinion in Otolaryngology, Head and Neck Surgery*, **12**, 76.

Brent RL. (1983) The effects of embryonic and fetal exposure to x-rays, microwaves and ultrasound. *Clinical Obstetrics and Gynecology*, **26**, 484, 1983.

Brewer M, Kueck A, Runowicz CD. (2011) Chemotherapy in pregnancy. *Clinical Obstetrics and Gynecology*, **54**, 602.

Bridges CC and Zalups RK. (2010) Transport of inorganic mercury and methylmercury in target tissues and organs. *Journal of Toxicology and Environmental Health*, **13**, 385.

Buekers TE and Thomas L. (1998) Chemotherapy in pregnancy. *Obstetrics and Gynecology*, **25**, 323–327.

Cardonic E and Lacobucci A. (2004) Use of chemotherapy during human pregnancy. *Lancet Oncology*, **5**, 283.

Cardoso da Silva HE, do Socorro Ramos Costa E, Quintão Medeiros AC, *et al.* (2016) Ameloblastoma during pregnancy. A case report. *Journal of Medical Case Reports*, **10**, 244.

Cariati P, Cabello-Serrano A, Monsalve-Iglesias F, *et al.* (2017). Juxtacortical mandibular chondrosarcoma during pregnancy. A case report. *Journal of Clinical and Experimental Dentistry*, **9**, e723.

Cengiz SB. (2007) The dental patient. Considerations for dental management and drug use. *Quintessence International*, **38**, 133.

Chen L and Suh BI. (2013) Bisphenol A in dental materials: a review. *JSM Dentistry*, **1**, 1004.

Cheung EJ, Wagner H, Botti JJ, *et al.* (2009) Advanced oral tongue cancer in a 22 year old pregnant woman. *Annals of Otology, Rhinology and Laryngology*, **118**, 21.

Chow VL, Chan JY, Ng RW, and Wei WI. (2008) Management of head and neck tumours during pregnancy. Case report and literature review. *Asian Journal of Surgery*, **31**, 199.

Cudney N, Ochs MW, Johnson J, *et al.* (2010) A unique presentation of a squamous cell carcinoma in a pregnant patient. *Quintessence International*, **41**, 581.

Da Costa EC, da Rosa LA, Batista DV. (2015) Fetus absorbed dose evaluation in head and neck radiotherapy procedures of pregnant patients. *Applied Radiation and Isotopes*, **100**, 11.

Dalla Torre D, Burtscher D, Hoefer D, *et al.* (2014) Odontogenic deep neck space infection as life-threatening condition in pregnancy. *Australian Dental Journal*, **59**, 375.

DeLair D, Bejarano PA, Peleg M, *et al.* (2007) Ameloblastic carcinosarcoma of the mandible arising in ameloblastic fibroma. a case report and review of the literature. *Oral Surgery, Oral Medicine, Oral Pathology, Oral Radiology and Endodontics*, **103**, 561.

Dellinger TM and Livingston MH. (2006) Pregnancy. Physiologic changes and considerations for dental patients. *Dental Clinics of North America*, **50**, 677.

Dennehy KC and Pian-Smith MC. (2000) Airway management of the parturient. *International Anesthesiology Clinics*, **38**, 147.

Doll R and Wakeford R. (1997) Risk of childhood cancer from fetal irradiation. *British Journal of Radiology*, **70**, 130.

Dumper J and Kerr P. (2005) Recurrent squamous cell carcinoma of the tongue in pregnancy. *Journal of Otolaryngology*, **34**, 242.

Edwards C, Yi CH, and Currie JL. (1995) Chorioamnionitis caused by Capnocytophaga. Case report. *American Journal of Obstetrics and Gynecology*, **173**, 244.

Eisig S and Carrao V. (2016) Management considerations to patients with endocrine diseases and the pregnant patient, in *Oral and Maxillofacial Surgery Secrets*, 3rd edn (eds A Abubaker, Din Lam, and K Benson), Mosby, St Louis, pp. 290–318.

Eliassen AM, Hauff SJ, Tang AL, *et al.* (2013) Head and neck squamous cell carcinoma in pregnant women. *Head and Neck*, **35**, 335.

Ferlito A, Devaney SL, Carbone A, *et al.* (1998) Pregnancy and malignant neoplasms of the head and neck. *Annals of Otology, Rhinology and Laryngology*, **107**, 991.

Flynn TR. (2014) Principles of management of odontogenic infections, in *Contemporary Oral and Maxillofacial Surgery*, 6th edn (eds JR Hupp, E Ellis E, and MTucker), Elsevier, Amsterdam, pp. 296–318.

Flynn TR and Susarla SM. (2007) Oral and maxillofacial surgery for the pregnant patient. *Oral and Maxillofacial Surgery Clinics of North America*, **19**, 207.

Fung Kee Fung K, Eason E, Crane J, *et al.* (2003) Prevention of Rh alloimmunization. *Journal of Obstetrics and Gynaecology Canada*, **25**, 765.

Garcia AG, Lopez JA, and Rey JMG. (2001) Squamous cell carcinoma of the maxilla during pregnancy. Report of case. *Journal of Oral and Maxillofacial Surgery*, **59**, 456.

Gawęda A, Jach E, Tomaszewski T, *et al.* (2011) Treatment of the follicular cyst of the mandible in a pregnant woman – a case study. *Journal of Pre-Clinical and Clinical Research*, **5**, 38.

Gordy FM, Holder R, O'Carroll MK, *et al.* (1996) Growth of an ameloblastoma during pregnancy. Opportunity lost? *Special Care in Dentistry*, **16**, 199.

Har-El G, Aroesty J, Shaha A, *et al.* (1994) Changing trends in deep neck abscess. A retrospective study of 110 patients. *Oral Surgery, Oral Medicine, Oral Pathology, Oral Radiology and Endodontics*, **77**, 446.

Hemalatha VT, Manigandan T, Sarumathi T, *et al.* (2013) Dental considerations in pregnancy – a critical review on the oral care. *Journal of Clinical and Diagnostic Research*, **7**, 948.

Herberts BG and Sandström J. (1957) Ameloblastoma occurring and recurring during pregnancies. *Acta Oto-Laryngologica*, **48**, 327.

Hilgenberg PB, Cunali RS, Bonotto D, *et al.* (2012) Temporomandibular disorders and pregnancy. *Revista Dor São Paulo*, **13**, 371.

Hill CC and Pickinpaugh J. (2008) Trauma and surgical emergencies in the obstetric patient. *Surgical Clinics of North America*, **88**, 421.

Hull SB and Bennett S. (2007) The pregnant trauma patient. Assessment and anesthetic management. *International Anesthesiology Clinics*, **45**, 1.

Hytten F. (1985) Blood volume changes in normal pregnancy. *Clinical Haematology*, **14**, 601.

Ibhawoh L and Enabulele J. (2015) Endodontic treatment of the pregnant patient. Knowledge, attitude and practices of dental residents. *Nigerian Medical Journal*, **56**, 311.

International Commission on Radiological Protection. (2000) Pregnancy and medical radiation. *Annals of the ICRP*, **30**, 1.

Jensen KS, Biggs KA, and Cardwell MS. (2015) Retropharyngeal abscess complicated by Prevotella buccae sepsis during pregnancy. A CASE REPORT. *Journal of Reproductive Medicine*, **60**, 87.

Jouppila R, Jouppila P, and Hollmen A. (1980) Laryngeal oedema as an obstetric anaesthesia complication. case reports. *Acta Anaesthesiologica Scandinavica*, **24**, 97.

Kal HB and Struikmans H. (2005) Radiotherapy during pregnancy. Fact and fiction. *Lancet Oncology*, **6**, 328.

Kanazawa I, Yamauchi M, Yanoi S, *et al.* (2009) Osteosarcoma in a pregnant patient with McCune–Albright syndrome. *Bone*, **45**, 603.

Kase KR, Svensson GK, Wolbarst AB, *et al.* (1983) Measurements of dose from secondary radiation outside a treatment field. *International Journal of Radiation Oncology Biology Physics*, **9**, 1177.

Khan I, Ansari MI, and Khan R. (2010) Oral surgery for the pregnant patient. *Heal Talk*, **3**, 31.

Klysik A, Kaszuba-Bartkowiak K, and Jurowski P. (2016) Axial length of the eyeball is important in secondary dislocation of the intraocular lens, capsular bag, and capsular tension ring complex. *Journal of Ophthalmology*, **1**, 6431438.

Koike T, Uehara S, Kobayashi H, *et al.* (2005) Squamous cell carcinoma experiences in two-year treatments. *Oral Oncology Extra*, **41**, 7.

Kurien S, Kattimani VS, Sriram R, *et al.* (2013) Management of pregnant patient in dentistry. *Journal of International Oral Health*, **5**, 88.

LaBauve JR, Long KN, Hack GD, *et al.* (2012) What every dentist should know about bisphenol A. *General Dentistry*, **60**, 424.

Lasaridis N, Tilaveridis I, and Karakasis D. (1996) Management of carcinoma of the tongue during pregnancy. Report of a case. *Journal of Oral and Maxillofacial Surgery*, **54**, 221.

Layton SA, Rintoul M, and Avery BS. (1992) Oral carcinoma in pregnancy. *British Journal of Oral and Maxillofacial Surgery*, **30**, 161.

LeResche L, Sherman JJ, Huggins K, *et al.* (2005) Musculoskeletal orofacial pain and other signs and symptoms of temporomandibular disorders during pregnancy. A prospective study. *Journal of Orofacial Pain*, **19**, 193.

Lin TI, Lin JC, Shih-Chu Ho E, *et al.* (2007) Nasopharyngeal carcinoma during pregnancy. *Obstetrics and Gynecology*, **46**, 423.

Lindbohm ML, Ylöstalo P, Sallmén M, *et al.* (2007) Occupational exposure in dentistry and miscarriage. *Occupational and Environmental Medicine*, **64**, 127.

Ling Yu Chow V, Yu Wai Chan J, Wai Man Ng Ri, *et al.* (2008) Management of head and neck tumours during pregnancy. Case report and literature review. *Asian Journal of Surgery*, **31**, 199.

Little JW. (2007) *Dental Management of the Medically Compromised Patient*, 7th edn, Mosby, St Louis, pp. 271–281.

Lloyd CJ, Paley MD, Penfold CN, *et al.* (2003) Microvascular free tissue transfer in the management of squamous cell carcinoma of the tongue during pregnancy. *British Journal of Oral and Maxillofacial Surgery*, **41**, 109.

Mayoral VA, Espinosa IA, and Montiel AJ. (2013) Association between signs and symptoms of temporomandibular disorders and pregnancy (case control study). *Acta Odontologica Latinoamericana*, **26**, 3.

McFarlane J, Parker B, Soeken K, *et al.* (1992) Assessing for abuse during pregnancy. Severity and frequency of injuries and associated entry into prenatal care. *Journal of the American Medical Association*, **267**, 3176.

Mendez-Figueroa H, Dahlke JD, Vrees RA, *et al.* (2013) Trauma in pregnancy. An updated systematic review. *American Journal of Obstetrics and Gynecology*, **209**, 1.

Mir O, Berveiller P, Ropert S, *et al.* (2008) Use of platinum derivatives during pregnancy. *Cancer*, **113**, 3069.

Morgan JA. (1925) Giant-cell sarcoma of the superior maxilla. *Laryngoscope*, **35**, 115.

Muench MV, Baschat AA, Reddy UM, *et al.* (2004) Kleihauer-Betke testing is important in all cases of maternal trauma. *Journal of Trauma*, **57**, 1094.

Murphy J, Berman D, Edwards SP, *et al.* (2016) Squamous cell carcinoma of the tongue during pregnancy. A case report and review of the literature. *Journal of Oral and Maxillofacial Surgery*, **74**, 2557.

Naseem M, Khurshid Z, Ali Khan H, *et al.* (2016) Oral health challenges in pregnant women. Recommendations for dental care professionals. *Saudi Journal for Dental Research*, **7**, 138.

Nuyttens JJ, Prado KL, Jenrette JM, *et al.* (2002) Fetal dose during radiotherapy. Clinical implementation and review of the literature. *Cancer/Radiotherapie*, **6**, 352.

O'Regan EM, Gibb DH, and Odell EW. (2001) Rapid growth of giant cell granuloma in pregnancy treated with calcitonin. *Oral Surgery, Oral Medicine, Oral Pathology, Oral Radiology and Endodontics*, **92**, 532.

Orlandi E, Zonca G, Pignoli E, *et al.* (2007) Postoperative radiotherapy for synovial sarcoma of the head and neck during pregnancy. Clinical and technical management and fetal dose estimates. *Tumori*, **93**, 452.

Osborn TM, Assael L, and Bell B. (2008) Deep space neck infection. Principles of surgical management. *Oral and Maxillofacial Surgery Clinics of North America*, **20**, 353.

Otsuka, Koji, Hamakawa H, Sumida T, and Tanioka H. (2001) Treatment of mandibular malignant fibrous histiocytoma during pregnancy. *Journal of Oral and Maxillofacial Surgery*, **59**, 220–224.

Palluch F, Lehmann M, Volz J, *et al.* (2011) The rapid growth of a pleomorphic adenoma of the parotid gland in the third trimester of pregnancy. *Journal of Medical Case Reports*, **5**, 141.

Patton LL and Glick M (eds) (2015) *The ADA Practical Guide to Patients with Medical Conditions*, Wiley Online Library, pp. 423–448.

Pearlman M and Faro S. (1990) Obstetric septic shock. A pathophysiologic basis for management. *Clinical Obstetrics and Gynecology*, **33**, 482.

Pearlman MD, Tintinalli JE, and Lorenz RP. (1990) A prospective controlled study of outcome after trauma during pregnancy. *American Journal of Obstetrics and Gynecology*, **162**, 1502.

Pereg D, Koren G, and Lishner M. (2008) Cancer in pregnancy. Gaps, challenges and solutions. *Cancer Treatment Review*, **34**, 302.

Petrone P and Marini CP. (2015) Trauma in pregnant patients. *Current Problems in Surgery*, **52**, 330.

Pirie M, Cook I, Linden G, *et al.* (2007) Dental manifestations of pregnancy. *Obstetrics and Gynaecology*, **9**, 21.

Poole GV, Martin JN, Perry KG, *et al.* (1996) Trauma in pregnancy. The role of interpersonal violence. *American Journal of Obstetrics and Gynecology*, **174**, 1873.

Prado KL, Nelson SJ, Nuyttens JJ, *et al.* (2000) Clinical implementation of the AAPM Task Group 36 recommendations on fetal dose from radiotherapy with photon beams. A head and neck irradiation case report. *Journal of Applied Clinical Medical Physics*, **1**, 1.

Puri A, Khadem P, Ahmed S, *et al.* (2012) Imaging of trauma in a pregnant patient. *Seminars in Ultrasound, CT and MR*, **33**, 37.

Rai B, Kaur J, and Kharb S. (2009) Pregnancy gingivitis and periodontitis and its systemic effect. *Internet Journal of Dental Science*, **6**.

Ramsay G, Paglia M, and Bourjeily G. (2013) When the heart stops. A review of cardiac arrest in pregnancy. *Journal of Intensive Care Medicine*, **28**, 204.

Reisner LS, Benumof JL, and Cooper SD. (1999) The difficult airway. Risk, prophylaxis and management, in *Obstetric Anesthesia*.

Principles and Practice (ed. DH Chestnut), Mosby, St Louis. pp. 590–620.

Schantz SP and Yu GP. (2002) Head and neck cancer incidence trends in young American, 1973–1997 with a special analysis for tongue cancer. *Archives of Otolaryngology, Head and Neck Surgery*, **128**, 268.

Sethi RK, Kozin ED, Fagenholz PJ, *et al.* (2014) Epidemiological survey of head and neck injuries and trauma in the United States. *Otolaryngology Head and Neck Surgery*, **151**, 776.

Shah AJ and Kilcline BA. (2003) Trauma in pregnancy. *Emergency Medicine Clinics of North America*, **21**, 615.

Shah KH, Simons RK, Holbrook T, *et al.* (1998) Trauma in pregnancy. Maternal and fetal outcomes. Journal of Trauma, **45**, 83.

Shen S, Xu L, Yin X, *et al.* (2011) A case of a squamous cell carcinoma of the tongue during pregnancy. *Oral Oncology*, **47**, 924.

Shessel BA, Portnof JE, Kaltman SI, *et al.* (2013) Dental treatment of the pregnant patient. Literature review and guidelines for the practicing clinician. *Today's FDA*, **25**, 26–29.

Shetty L, Shete A, and Gupta AA. (2015) Pregnant oral and maxillofacial patient – Catch 22 situation. *Dentistry*, **5**, 9.

Shibuya H, Saiot M, Horiuchi JI, *et al.* (1987) Treatment of malignant head and neck tumors during pregnancy – a report of 3 cases. *Acta Oncologica*, **26**, 237.

Shimanovich I, Skrobek C, Rose C, *et al.* (2002) Pemphigoid gestationis with predominant involvement of oral mucous membranes and IgA autoantibodies targeting the C-terminus of BP180. *Journal of the American Academy of Dermatology*, **47**, 780.

Shinozaki Y, Jinbu Y, Kusama M, *et al.* (2004) A case report of adenomatoid odontogenic tumor arising in a pregnant woman. *Oral Medicine and Pathology*, **9**, 31.

Siepermann M, Koscielniak E, Dantonello T, *et al.* (2012) Oral low-dose chemotherapy. Successful treatment of an alveolar rhabdomyosarcoma during pregnancy. *Pediatric Blood and Cancer*, **58**, 104.

Silasi M, Cardenas I, Racicot K, *et al.* (2015) Viral infections during pregnancy. *American Journal of Reproductive Immunology*, **73**, 199.

Smith JA, Gaikwad A, Mosley S, *et al.* (2014) Utilization of an ex vivo human placental perfusion model to predict potential fetal exposure to carboplatin during pregnancy. *American Journal of Obstetrics and Gynecology*, **210**, 275.

Solak Ö, Turhan-Haktanir N, Köken G, *et al.* (2009) Prevalence of temporomandibular disorders in pregnancy. *European Journal of General Medicine*, **6**, 223.

Sperry JL, Casey BM, McIntire DD, *et al.* (2006) Long-term fetal outcomes in pregnant trauma patients. *American Journal of Surgery*, **192**, 715.

Stone K. (1999) Trauma in the obstetric patient. *Obstetric and Gynecology Clinics of North America*, **26**, 459.

Stoval M, Blackwell CR, Cundiff J, *et al.* (1995) Fetal dose from radiotherapy with photon beams. Report of AAPM Radiation Therapy Committee Task Group No 36. *Medical Physics*, **22**, 63.

Tagliabue M, Elrefaey SH, Peccatori F, *et al.* (2016) Tongue cancer during pregnancy. Surgery and more, a multidisciplinary challenge. *Critical Reviews of Oncology and Hematology*, **98**, 1.

Takalkar AM, Khandelwal A, Lokitz S, *et al.* (2011) 18 F-FDG PET in pregnancy and fetal radiation dose estimates. *Journal of Nuclear Medicine*, **52**, 1035.

Teoh M, Clark CH, Wood K, *et al.* (2011) Volumetric modulate arc therapy. A review of current literature and clinical use in practice. *British Journal of Radiology*, **84**, 967.

Terada T, Uwa N, Sagawa K, *et al.* (2015) A case of tongue carcinoma resection and reconstruction with microsurgical free flap during pregnancy. *Nihon Jibiinkoka Gakkai Kaiho*, **118**, 46.

Terenzi V, Cassoni A, della Monaca M, *et al.* (2016) Oral cancer during pregnancy. *Oral Oncology*, **59**, 1.

Tocaciu S, Robinson BW, and Sambrook BJ. (2017) Severe odontogenic infection in pregnancy. A timely reminder. *Australian Dental Journal*, **62**, 98.

Triunfo S and Scambia G. (2014) Cancer in pregnancy. diagnosis, treatment and neonatal outcome. *Minerva Ginecologica*, **66**, 325.

Tubbs RS, Shoja MM, Loukas M, *et al.* (2010) William Henry Battle and Battle's sign. Mastoid ecchymosis as an indicator of basilar skull fracture. *Journal of Neurosurgery*, **112**, 186.

Turner M and Aziz SR. (2002) Management of the pregnant oral and maxillofacial surgery patient. *Journal of Oral and Maxillofacial Surgery*, **60**, 1479.

Tweddale CJ. (2006) Trauma during pregnancy. *Critical Care Nursing Quarterly*, **29**, 53.

Unsworth JD, Baldwin A, Byrd L. (2013) Systemic lupus erythematosus, pregnancy and carcinoma of the tongue. BMJ Case Reports, bcr-2013-008864.

Voulgaris E, Pentheroudakis G, and Pavlidis N. (2011) Cancer and pregnancy. A comprehensive review. *Journal of Surgical Oncology*, **20**, e175.

Wang B, Gao BL, Xu GP, *et al.* (2014) Images of deep neck space infection and the clinical significance. *Acta Radiologica*, **55**, 945.

Wazir S, Khan M, Mansoor N, *et al.* (2013) Odontogenic facial space infections in pregnancy – a study. *Pakistan Oral and Dental Journal*, **33**, 17.

Wise RA, Polito AJ, and Krishnan V. (2006) Respiratory physiologic changes in pregnancy. *Immunology and Allergy Clinics of North America*, **26**, 1.

Wolf EJ, Mallozzi A, Rodis JF, *et al.* (1992) The principal pregnancy complications resulting in preterm birth in singleton and twin gestations. *Journal of Maternal and Fetal Medicine*, **14**, 206.

Yamoah KK, Lindow S, and Karsaia L. (2009) Large epulis in pregnancy. *Journal of Obstetrics and Gynaecology*, **29**, 761.

Yokoshima K, Nakamizo M, Sakanushi A, *et al.* (2012) Surgical management of tongue cancer during pregnancy. *Auris Nasus Larynx*, **39**, 428.

Yoruk O, Ucuncu H, Gursan N, *et al.* (2009) Sinonasal Burkitt lymphoma presenting as a nasal polyposis in a pregnant woman. *Journal of Craniofacial Surgery*, **20**, 1059.

Zemlickis D, Lishner M, Degendorfer P, *et al.* (1992) Fetal outcome after in utero exposure to cancer chemotherapy. *Archives of Internal Medicine*, **152**, 573.

7

Postnatal Considerations
Kyriaki C. Marti

A very important part of the postnatal period is the time of breastfeeding. It is essential that the woman who breastfeeds her infant for a shorter or longer period of time should be aware of her nutrition, psychologic, and physical health as she is directly responsible for the newborn baby. Breast milk has unique properties that make it the only source of nutrition a healthy infant requires for about the first 6 months of life. Numerous studies have documented the health benefits of breastfeeding for the infant and the mother. These health benefits are listed in Boxes 7.1 and 7.2.

Note: The health provider should be aware of *postpartum preeclampsia*. It is described as a rare condition that occurs when a woman has high blood pressure and excess protein in her urine soon after childbirth. Most cases develop within 48 hours of childbirth but, according to Clark (2014), it may present up to 6 weeks after childbirth (see also "Preeclampsia" in Chapter 9).

Medical Contraindications to Breastfeeding

- Maternal illness (e.g., HIV, human T cell lymphotropic virus type I or type II, active herpes simplex lesions on the breast, acute H1N1 infection, Ebola virus and brucellosis, active untreated tuberculosis or active varicella, use of drugs of abuse, antimetabolites, chemotherapeutic agents, or radioisotopes).
- Infants who have type 1 galactosemia should not be breastfed; some other inborn errors of metabolism may require feeding modification.

Breastfeeding and Infant Oral Health

From an infant oral health standpoint, there is an ongoing discussion on two issues regarding the potential oral sequelae of breastfeeding:

- the potential of development of malocclusion
- early childhood caries (ECC).

The current literature indicates that there is no strong evidence that an association exists between breastfeeding and malocclusion or ECC. The consensus among health organizations (AAP, APHA, ACOG, AAFP, ACN-M, AND) is that infants should be breastfed exclusively for about the first 6 months of life, and that breastfeeding should continue for at least the first year of the child's life.

Box 7.1 Breastfeeding health benefits: infant.

Acute otitis media (AOM):	Risk of AOM two- fold for exclusively formula-fed infants compared with those breastfed exclusively for 3–6 months
Gastroenteritis/diarrhea:	Risk of diarrhea-related mortality (infant age 0 through 5 months), higher in partially breastfed than in exclusively breastfed infants
Respiratory tract infections (RTIs):	Risk of being hospitalized for RTIs (otherwise healthy infants), lower among those breastfed exclusively for 4 months compared with formula-fed infants
Necrotizing enterocolitis (NEC):	Absolute risk difference of 5% found between breastfed infants and those who were not
Leukemia:	Risk of acute lymphocytic and myelogenous leukemia significantly reduced among infants breastfed for more than 6 months
Sudden infant death syndrome (SIDS):	SIDS risk for breastfed infants lower than those who were never breastfed
Asthma:	Risk of asthma lower in infants with no family history of asthma, breastfed exclusively for at least 3 months, compared with infants who were not breastfed
Obesity:	Risk of childhood obesity lower among breastfed infants compared to those who were formula fed
Diabetes mellitus type 2 (DMT2):	Risk for DMT2 later in life lower in breastfeeding compared to formula feeding

---

Box 7.2 Breastfeeding health benefits: mother.

Postpartum bleeding and hemorrhage risk:	Reduced
Lactational amenorrhea and suppression of ovulation:	Provide time to recover fully from pregnancy and childbirth, as well as a nonpharmacological method of family planning
Breast cancer:	Each additional year of breastfeeding reduces breast cancer risk by 4.3%
Ovarian cancer:	Risk decreased by 2% for each month of breastfeeding and was also lower in those who had ever breastfed compared with those who had never breastfed
Multiple sclerosis (MS):	Mothers who breastfeed longer may be at lower risk of developing MS

In an effort to prevent ECC, it has been recommended that oral hygiene should begin as soon as the first tooth appears and that the consumption of sugary beverages be minimized.

The presence of natal teeth is also an issue that requires attention. Their extraction may be warranted if they traumatize the nipples and areolae during breastfeeding, interfere with suckling, cause traumatic sublingual ulceration (Riga–Fede disease) resulting in feeding refusal, are supernumerary and pose a risk of being swallowed or aspirated. Riga–Fede disease was named after two Italian physicians (Antonio Riga and Francesco Fede). Riga's first report on the condition was published in 1881. Fede, who is considered the father of Italian pediatrics, reported additional cases enriched with histopathogy in 1891.

Procedures and Medications During Breastfeeding

Dental procedures, such as prevention and treatment of dental caries, and periodontal disease as well as endodontics, orthodontics, and prosthetics, can be safely performed during lactation and breastfeeding. Oral and maxillofacial procedures that do not require lengthy hospitalization and prolonged recovery can also be performed during lactation and breastfeeding. Implant placement, orthognathic, and cosmetic procedures can be delayed until after the cessation of breastfeeding, but surgery for infections regardless of origin, trauma, benign locally aggressive and malignant tumors and associated reconstructive procedures, although they will require interruption of breastfeeding, should be performed without delay. If maternal illness causes separation, assistance with maintaining lactation should be provided. When separation is inevitable, stored maternal milk or formula can replace breastfeeding (existing guidelines for breastmilk storage should be implemented).

Local Anesthesia

According to the AAP, lidocaine is considered to be safe for the breastfeeding patient. Lidocaine is the most commonly used and best studied local anesthetic in pregnancy and lactation while other amide or hybrid anesthetics may also be used (although they present a slightly higher association with side effects). Ester anesthetics are avoided due to higher risk for allergic reactions.

It is essential that dentists follow administration guidelines carefully. As dental care is often deferred immediately after giving birth, it is important to adhere to best techniques (meticulous aspiration to avoid intravascular administration, correct positioning of the needle, and limitation of local anesthetic to safe dosages). The use of vasoconstriction is considered beneficial by some authors, since it decreases local anesthetic toxicity, provided that a proper aspiration technique ensures prevention of intravascular injection. The epinephrine contained in a local anesthetic solution, if injected intravascularly, has the potential to worsen the maternal hypercoagulable state that can last for 6–12 weeks post partum, through an increase in thrombin and factor VIII levels and activation of the coagulation cascade. Although an extremely low dose of exogenous epinephrine vasoconstrictor enters the circulation, the possible effect on a hypercoagulable patient should be considered.

Moreover, lactating patients may be treated with anticoagulants due to higher risk of thrombosis during lactation compared to pregnancy, especially during the first 6–12 weeks after labor, as mentioned above. Boer *et al.* (2007) presented the hypothesis that the increased tissue factor (TF) levels activate coagulation and therefore it should be borne in mind that the use of local anesthesia can lead to hematoma formation in a patient on low molecular heparin therapy.

Another issue to consider is that during the postnatal period, postpartum depression is seen in approximately 13% of women and often remains untreated. Treatment includes individual psychotherapy and antidepressant drug therapy. Maternal antidepressant therapy carries risks for nursing infants and the risks and benefits of treatment are carefully weighed for each individual patient. Patients receiving antidepressant therapy are at risk of developing xerostomia and orthostatic hypotension. Dentists must take precautions during the use of vasoconstrictors because of their interactions particularly with tricyclic antidepressants and nonselective beta-adrenergic blockers. It is also prudent to use adrenergic vasoconstrictors cautiously in patients with postpartum hyperthyroidism.

The safety of local anesthetics during breastfeeding is summarized in Table 7.1.

Nitrous Oxide, Oral Sedation, Procedural Intravenous Sedation and General Anesthesia

Maternal procedural intravenous sedation (PIVS) and general anesthesia rarely contraindicate breastfeeding. Most agents used for PIVS and general anesthesia have short half-lives and clear the maternal circulation rapidly. There is no need to delay breastfeeding after general anesthesia for a procedure done within the first 2–3 days post partum (e.g., tubal ligation) because the amount of colostrum is too small to carry a significant quantity of the anesthetic agents. For surgical procedures done later, the decision about resuming breastfeeding depends on the condition of the infant. Mothers of healthy term neonates can resume breastfeeding once they are awake and able to hold the infant. In the case of a preterm or otherwise compro-

mised neonate, pumping and discarding the milk for 12–24 hours after the procedure may be warranted. The safety of nitrous oxide, oral and intravenous sedation, and anesthetic drugs is summarized in Table 7.2.

Prescription and OTC Medications During Breastfeeding

The health provider needs to be aware of the medications that are allowed during lactation and breastfeeding as well as being prepared to educate the mother about potential side effects of drugs and chemicals excreted in breast milk.

The numbers of breastfeeding mothers are increasing in the US, as three out of every four new mothers in the US now start out breastfeeding. However, rates of breastfeeding at 6 and 12 months, as well as rates of

Table 7.1 Local anesthetic selection during breastfeeding.

	Safety in breastfeeding
Local anesthetic (injectable)	
Lidocaine	Safe
Prilocaine	Safe
Articaine	Caution
Bupivacaine	Safe
Mepivacaine	Safe
Local anesthetic (topical)	
Lidocaine	Safe
Lidocaine + prilocaine	Safe
Benzocaine	Caution*
Tetracaine	Caution*

*Can cause acquired methemoglobenemia.

Table 7.2 Nitrous oxide, oral sedation, IV sedation and general anesthesia during breastfeeding.

	Safety in breastfeeding
Intravenous drugs	
Fentanyl	Safe
Midazolam	Safe
Etomidate	Safe
Propofol	Safe
Ketamine	Caution – limited data
Oral sedatives	
Lorazepam	Safe (short half-life than other benzodiazepines)
Oxazepam	
Nitrous oxide	Safe
General anesthetics	
Volatile agents	Considered safe (rapid elimination, poor bioavailability)
Neuromuscular blocking agents	Considered safe (relatively large size, low lipid solubility, polarized nature)
Opioid and muscle relaxant reversals	Safe

exclusive breastfeeding at 3 and 6 months, remain stagnant and low. This is mainly due to the American Academy of Pediatrics (AAP) position paper which emphasized the value of breastfeeding as the best nutritional mode for infants in their first 6 months of life. This paper led to the recommendation that most US infants be breastfed exclusively for about the first 6 months of life, and that breastfeeding should continue for at least the first year of the child's life. This recommendation resulted in high rates of breastfeeding as well as increased concerns about the health needs of infants among parents, physicians, dentists, pharmacists, nurses, and other health professionals.

An important limitation of studies on the safety of medications during lactation and breastfeeding is the fact that most studies on human lactation were carried out on animals, due to the evident ethical considerations. According to Donaldson and Goodchild (2012), the general rule that can be applied for the breastfeeding patient is that "if a drug is considered acceptable for use during pregnancy, it is usually reasonable to continue its use during breastfeeding." However, there are important exceptions to that recommendation related to:

- molecular weight of substances
- metabolism of the drug in the neonatal circulation.

Analgesics

Table 7.3 summarizes the safety of prescription analgesics during breastfeeding.

Acetaminophen remains the analgesic of choice provided that dosage does not reach hepatotoxicity levels. Of the nonsteroidal antiinflammatory drugs (NSAIDs), ibuprofen is the preferred choice because it has poor transfer into milk and has been well studied in children. Long half-life NSAIDs such as naproxen, sulindac, and piroxicam can accumulate in the infant with prolonged use.

Potent prescription analgesics such as oxycodone and hydrocodone should be utilized with caution during lactation. According to

Table 7.3 Analgesic selection during breastfeeding

	Safety during breastfeeding
Acetaminophen	Safe
Aspirin	Caution
Ibuprofen	Safe
Codeine	Safe
Hydrocodone	Caution
Oxycodone	Caution
Morphine	Safe

Sachs (2013), the use of any oral narcotic during lactation can cause drowsiness, central nervous system depression, and even death to the neonate. In particular, newborns are very sensitive to even a small dose of narcotic analgesics.

Furthermore, elimination of a drug such as oxycodone and hydrocodone is decreased in infants, while interindividual variability exists, and these drugs are considered dangerous for newborns. Oxycodone is detected in human breast milk and in a study by Seaton *et al.* (2007), mothers receiving oxycodone for surgical pain control (cesarean section) had measureable milk and serum oxycodone levels at 24, 48, and 72 hours post partum. Therefore, use should be controlled to a few days and a limited dose (30 mg daily for maximum maternal uptake). Concurrently, the infant should be monitored for drowsiness, increased sleepiness, breathing pattern, and normal weight gain, as well as other developmental milestones. Other nonnarcotic agents are preferred during this period.

Recently, the FDA published a *strengthened Warning* to breastfeeding mothers on the use of opioid medications during lactation: "Breastfeeding is not recommended when taking codeine or tramadol medicines due to the risk of serious adverse reactions in breastfed infants. These can include excess sleepiness, difficulty breastfeeding, or serious breathing problems that could result in death" (FDA 2017).

Antibiotics

The use of most antibiotics is considered compatible with breastfeeding. Penicillins, aminopenicillins, clavulanic acid, cephalosporins, macrolides, and metronidazole at dosages at the low end of the recommended range are considered appropriate for lactating women. Fluoroquinolones should not be administered as first-line treatment, but

if they are indicated, breastfeeding should not be interrupted because the risk of adverse effects is low and the risks are justified. Safety of antibiotics during breastfeeding is summarized in Table 7.4.

Corticosteroids

Corticosteroids are generally considered safe for use by breastfeeding mothers. A

Table 7.4 Antibiotic selection during breastfeeding.

	Safety in breastfeeding
Penicillins	
Penicillin (VK,G)	Safe
Amoxicillin	Safe
Amoxicillin + clavulanic acid	Safe
Cephalosporins	
All generations	Safe
Carbapenems	
Doripenem	Safe
Ertapenem	Safe
Meropenem	Safe
Imipenem-cilastatin	Safe
Monobactams	
Aztreonam	Safe
Glycopeptides	
Vancomycin	Safe
Macrolides	
Erythromycin (base form)*	Safe
Azithromycin	Safe
Clarithromycin	Safe
Tetracyclines	
Tetracycline	Unsafe
Minocycline	Unsafe
Doxycycline	Unsafe

	Safety in breastfeeding
Aminoglycocides	
Amikacin	Safe
Gentamycin	Safe
Streptomycin	Safe
Tobramycin	Safe
Fluoroquinolones	
Ciprofloxacin	Unsafe
Norfloxacin	Unsafe
Ofloxacin	Unsafe
Enoxacin	Unsafe
Miscellaneous antibiotics	
Clindamycin	Safe
Metronidazole	Avoid – gives milk unpleasant taste
Antifungals	
Nystatin	Safe
Clotrimazole	Safe
Griseofulvin	No data
Ketoconazole	Unsafe
Fluconazole	Safe
Amphotericin B	No data
Antivirals	
Acyclovir	Safe
Valacyclovir	Safe
Famciclovir	No data
Penciclovir	No data
Chlorhexidine gluconate	Safe

* The estolate form of erythromycin is contraindicated
Source: www.drugs.com

small amount of the steroid passes to the infant, but repeated trials and clinical reports have shown no negative side effects. However, betamethasone, dexamethasone, hydrocortisone, and triamcinolone have not been well studied during breastfeeding after systemic or topical use (Table 7.5). Systemic administration of these steroids is best avoided in favor of one of the shorter-acting and better studied alternatives.

OTC medications

Even though most OTC medications are safe during breastfeeding (Table 7.6), precautions to lower any potential risk even further include the following.

- The lowest possible dose should be used and for the shortest possible time.
- Extra-strength formulas should be avoided.
- Sustained-release preparations and medications indicated for use only once or twice a day should be avoided. These are usually long-acting drugs and remain in maternal circulation and breastmilk much longer than drugs that need to be taken more frequently.
- When possible, single-ingredient preparations rather than multi-symptom formulas should be used.

Table 7.5 Corticosteroid selection during breastfeeding.

	Safety in breastfeeding
Betamethasone	Caution – limited data
Dexamethasone	Caution – limited data
Hydrocortisone	Caution – limited data
Methylprednisolone	Safe
Prednisolone	Safe
Prednisone	Safe
Triamcinolone	Caution – limited data

Source: www.drugs.com

Pharmacologic Substances Used in the Treatment of Keratocystic Odontogenic Tumor

- Carnoy's solution: there are no data on the safety of the topical application of Carnoy's solution for the treatment of a KOT if the lesion requires surgical treatment during the period of breastfeeding.
- 5-Fluorouracil (5-FU): there are no data as to the systemic absorption of 5-FU, which was recently introduced as part of the surgical management of KOT. Although it is believed that topical 5-FU applied away from the breast should pose negligible risk for the breastfed infant, inference cannot be made as to its presence and concentration in maternal milk when it is applied locally in the treatment of KOT.

Diagnostic Imaging During Breastfeeding

In the postpartum period, confusion on the safety of imaging modalities can result in either the unnecessary avoidance of important diagnostic tests or the unwarranted interruption of breastfeeding for the nursing mother. According to the American College of Obstetricians and Gynecologists (ACOG), Committee on Obstetric Practice, ultrasonography and magnetic resonance imaging are not associated with risk, and therefore they are the imaging techniques of choice for this period, "only when used prudently and only when its use is expected to answer a relevant clinical question or provide medical benefit to the patient."

Conventional X-rays

There is no risk to lactation from external sources of ionizing radiation used for diagnostic imaging.

Computed Tomography Scans

All concerns are limited to examinations requiring the use of contrast agents in the postnatal period. Oral contrast agents are not absorbed by the patient and therefore do not cause any real or theoretical harm. The

Table 7.6 Safety of OTC medications during breastfeeding.

	Safety in breastfeeding		Safety in breastfeeding
Antihistamines		Lansoprazole	Safe
Diphenhydramine	Safe	Aluminum hydroxide	Safe
Brompheniramine	Safe	Calcium carbonate	Safe
Chlorpheniramine	Safe	Magnesium carbonate/ hydroxide	Safe
Pheniramine	Safe		
Cetirizine	Safe	**Antiflatulent**	
Loratadine	Safe	Simethicone	Safe
Fexofenadine	Safe	**Antidiarrheals**	
Expectorant		Bismuth subsalicylate	Avoid (salicylate content)
Guaifenesin	Avoid; no data, alcohol content	Loperamide	Safe
Nonnarcotic antitussive		**Laxatives**	
Dextromethorphan	Avoid; no data, alcohol content	Mineral oil	Safe
		Castor oil	Avoid; no data
Antacids		Polyethylene glycol 3350	Avoid; no data
Cimetidine	Caution (potential for hepatic enzyme inhibition)	**Decongestants**	
		Pseudoephedrine	Avoid (irritability in infants, decrease in maternal milk production)
Famotidine	Safe		
Nizatidine	Safe		
Ranitidine	Safe	Oxymetazoline	Safe (decongestant of choice)
Omeprazole	Safe		
Esomeprazole	Safe		
Rabeprazole	Avoid; no data		

Source: www.drugs.com

use of intravenous contrast media aids in CT imaging is recommended for better visualization of soft or vascular tissues.

Traditionally, advice to lactating women was to discontinue breastfeeding for 24 hours after intravenous administration of iodinated contrast agents. However, recent literature suggests that breastfeeding can be continued without interruption after use of iodinated contrast media.

Magnetic Resonance Imaging
Breastfeeding should not be interrupted after gadolinium contrast administration (for MRI). Literature has shown that the water solubility of gadolinium-based agents limits their excretion into breast milk. The 2016 Committee Opinion of the ACOG states that:

"Less than 0.04% of the intravascular dose of gadolinium contrast is excreted in breast milk within 24 hours, and the infant absorbs less than 1% from this amount in their GI tract. No reports of harm where also found relative to any unchelated gadolinium excreted in the breast milk and reaching potentially the newborn."

Nuclear Medicine Imaging (Ventilation-Perfusion Scan, Thyroid, Bone or Renal Scan)

The use of a radioisotope-containing agent is required. The radioisotope commonly used in pregnancy is technetium 99 m which has a half -life of 6 hours at a dose of 5 mGy (indicated dose during pregnancy). Radionuclide compounds are excreted into breast milk in various concentrations and for various periods of time, while rates of excretion vary among patients. The lactating woman should have consultations with experts on breastfeeding and nuclear medicine to identify potential recommended uses of radionuclide agents and to decide about the use of nuclear medicine imaging during lactation, due to increased risk of harm to the neonate. Risks and benefits should always be thoroughly discussed with the patient.

Positron Emission Tomography Scan

Hicks *et al.* (2001) studied the pattern of uptake and excretion of 18 F-FDG in the lactating breast and concluded that "there is little secretion of activity into breast milk, and that higher radiation dose is received by the infant from close contact with the breast than from ingestion of radioactive milk." In patients reluctant to discontinue breastfeeding, expression of breast milk and bottlefeeding by a third party could help to minimize radiation exposure to the infant. Alternatively, Jamar *et al.* (2013) suggest that the infant can be breastfed 12 hours after maternal ingestion of 18 F-FDG.

References

American College of Obstetricians and Gynecologists Committee on Obstetric Practice (2016) Committee Opinion No. 656. Guidelines for Diagnostic Imaging During Pregnancy and Lactation. *Obstetrics and Gynecology*, **127**, e75.

Boer K, den Hollander IA, Meijers JCM, and Levi M. (2007) Tissue factor-dependent blood cogulation is enhanced following delivery irrespective of the mode of delivery. *Journal of Thrombosis and Haemostasis*, **5**, 2415.

Clark TP. (2014) Late-onset postpartum preeclampsia. A case study. *Nurse Practitioner*, **39**, 34.

Donaldson M and Goodchild JH. (2012) Pregnancy, breast-feeding and drugs used in dentistry. *Journal of the American Dental Association*, **143**, 858.

FDA (2015) FDA Drug Safety Communication. FDA has reviewed possible risks of pain medicine use during pregnancy. Available online at: www.fda.gov/Drugs/DrugSafety/ucm429117.htm (accessed 23 October 2017).

FDA (2017) Available online at: www.fda.gov/Drugs/DrugSafety/ucm549679.htm (accessed 23 October 2017).

Hicks RJ, Binns D, and Stabin MG. (2001) Pattern of uptake and excretion of 18F-FDG in the lactating breast. *Journal of Nuclear Medicine*, **42**, 1238.

Jamar F, Buscombe J, Chiti A, *et al.* (2013) EANM/SNMMI guideline for 18F-FDG use in inflammation and infection. *Journal of Nuclear Medicine*, **54**, 646.

Sachs HC. (2013) The transfer of drugs and therapeutics into human breast milk, an updated on selected topics. Committee of Drugs. *Pediatrics*, **132**, 796.

Seaton S, Reeves M, and McLean S, (2007) Oxycodone as a component of multimodal analgesia for lactating mothers after Caesarean section, Relationships between maternal plasma, breast milk and neonatal plasma levels. *Australia and New Zealand Journal of Obstetrics and Gynaecology*, **47**, 181.

Further Reading

[no authors listed] (1994) AAP issues policy statement on the transfer of drugs and other chemicals into human milk. *American Family Physician*, **49**, 1527.

AAFP position paper on breastfeeding. Available online at: www.aafp.org/about/policies/all/breastfeeding-support.html (accessed 23 October 2017).

Adam A, Dixon AK, Gillard JH, and Schafer-Prokop CM (eds) (2015) *Grainger and Allison's Diagnostic Radiology – A Textbook of Medical Imaging*, 6th edn, Churchill Livingstone/Elsevier New York, pp. 76–135.

Azizi F and Amouzegar A. (2011) Management of hyperthyroidism during pregnancy and lactation. *European Journal of Endocrinology*, **164**, 871.

Bar-Oz B, Bulkowstein M, Benyamini L, *et al.* (2003) Use of antibiotic and analgesic drugs during lactation. *Drug Safety*, **26**, 925.

Cengiz SB. (2007) The dental patient. Considerations for dental management and drug use. *Quintessence International*, **38**, 133.

Chen MM, Coakley FV, Kaimal A, *et al.* (2008) Guidelines for computed tomography and magnetic resonance imaging use during pregnancy and lactation. *Obstetrics and Gynecology*, **112**, 333.

Cleveland Clinic. *Over-the-Counter Medications and Breastfeeding.* Available online at: my.clevelandclinic.org/health/articles/over-the-counter-medications-and-breastfeeding (accessed 23 October 2017).

Cobb B, Liu R, Valentine E, *et al.* (2015) Breastfeeding after anesthesia. A review for anesthesia providers regarding the transfer of medications into breast milk. *Translational Perioperative and Pain Medicine*, **1**, 1.

Dashow JE, McHugh JB, Braun TM, *et al.* (2015) Significantly decreased recurrence rates in keratocystic odontogenic tumor with simple enucleation and curettage using Carnoy's versus modified Carnoy's solution. *Journal of Oral and Maxillofacial Surgery*, **73**, 2132.

Fayans EP, Stuart HR, Carsten D, *et al.* (2010) Local anesthetic use in the pregnant and postpartum patient. *Dental Clinics of North America*, **54**, 697.

Flynn TR and Susarla SM. (2007) Oral and maxillofacial surgery for the pregnant patient. *Oral and Maxillofacial Surgery Clinics of North America*, **19**, 207.

Gjelsteen AC, Ching BH, Meyermann MW, *et al.* (2008) CT, MRI, PET, PET/CT, and ultrasound in the evaluation of obstetric and gynecologic patients. *Surgical Clinics of North America*, **88**, 361.

Gjerdingen D. (2003) The effectiveness of various postpartum depression treatments and the impact of antidepressant drugs on nursing infants. *Journal of the American Board of Family Practice*, **16**, 372.

Groen RS, Bae JY, and Lim KJ. (2012) Fear of the unknown, ionizing radiation exposure during pregnancy. *American Journal of Obstetrics and Gynecology*, **206**, 456.

Horner K, Islam M, Flygare L, *et al.* (2009) Basic principles for use of dental cone beam computed tomography: consensus guidelines of the European Academy of Dental and Maxillofacial Radiology. *Dentomaxillofacial Radiology*, **38**, 187.

Keene JJ, Galasko GT, and Land MF. (2003) Antidepressant use in psychiatry and medicine, importance for dental practice. *Journal of the American Dental Association*, **134**, 71.

Langer-Gould A, Smith JB, Hellwig K, *et al.* (2017) Breastfeeding, ovulatory years, and risk of multiple sclerosis. *Neurology*, **89**, 563.

Ledderhof NJ, Caminiti MF, Bradley G, *et al.* (2017) Topical 5-fluorouracil is a novel targeted therapy for the keratocystic odontogenic tumor. *Journal of Oral and Maxillofacial Surgery*, **75**, 514.

Peccatori FA, Giovannetti E, Pistilli B, *et al.* (2012) "The only thing I know is that I know nothing": 5-fluorouracil in human milk. *Annals of Oncology*, **23**, 543.

Pokela ML, Anttila E, Seppala T, *et al.* (2005) Marked variation in oxycodone pharmacokinetics in infants. *Paediatric Anaesthesia*, **15**, 560.

Salone LR, Vann Jr WF, and Dee DL. (2013) Breastfeeding. An overview of oral and general health benefits. *Journal of the American Dental Association*, **144**, 143.

Scarfe WC, Levin MD, Gane D, *et al.* (2009) Use of cone beam computed tomography in endodontics. *International Journal of Dentistry*, Article ID 634567. DOI: 10.1155/2009/634567.

So M, Bozzo P, Inoue M, *et al.* (2010) Safety of antihistamines during pregnancy and lactation. *Canadian Family Physician*, **56**, 427.

Spencer JP, Gonzalez III LS, and Barnhart DJ. (2001) Medications in the breast-feeding mother. *American Family Physician*, **64**, 119.

Suresh L and Radfar L. (2004) Pregnancy and lactation. *Oral Surgery, Oral Medicine, Oral Pathology, Oral Radiology and Endodontics*, **97**, 672.

Tremblay E, Therasse E, Thomassin-Naggara I, *et al.* (2012) Quality initiatives, guidelines for use of medical imaging during pregnancy and lactation. *Radiographics*, **32**, 897.

Turner M and Aziz SR. (2002) Management of the pregnant oral and maxillofacial surgery patient. *Journal of Oral and Maxillofacial Surgery*, **60**, 1479.

Wang P, Chong S, Kielar A, *et al.* (2012) Imaging of pregnant and lactating patients, Part 1, evidence-based review and recommendations. *American Journal of Roentgenology*, **198**, 778.

White SC, Heslop EW, Hollender LG, *et al.* (2001) Parameters of radiologic care. An official report of the American Academy of Oral and Maxillofacial Radiology. *Oral Surgery, Oral Medicine, Oral Pathology, Oral Radiology and Endodontics*, **91**, 498.

Yagiela JA. (1999) Adverse drug interactions in dental practice: interactions associated with vasoconstrictors, part V of a series. *Journal of the American Dental Association*, **130**, 701.

8

Basic Life Support (BLS) and Advanced Cardiac Life Support (ACLS) in Pregnancy

Kyriaki C. Marti

Cardiac Arrest in Pregnancy

Incidence

The incidence of maternal cardiac arrest reported in the literature has been variable; it has been cited as 1 in 30 000 pregnancies. Recent data from the US Nationwide Inpatient Sample suggest that cardiac arrest occurs in 1:12 000 admissions for delivery. Globally, 800 maternal deaths occur daily. Maternal mortality trends in the United States reported by the CDC show a steady increase from 7.2 deaths per 100 000 live births in 1987 to 17.8 deaths per 100 000 live births in 2009.

Causes of cardiac arrest during pregnancy can be nonobstetric or obstetric (Box 8.1).

BLS

It is essential that the anatomic and physiologic changes during pregnancy as well as the gestational age are taken into consideration for effective management of maternal cardiac arrest. The AHA introduced certain modifications to the BLS protocol in the Scientific Statement on Cardiac Arrest in Pregnancy released in 2015.

Chest Compressions

Old Recommendations
- Chest compressions are performed with the patient in a 15–30° tilted position.
- Hands are placed slightly higher on the sternum.

New Recommendations
- Chest compressions are performed with the patient in supine position.
- Hands are placed over the lower third of the sternum (no change from existing protocol) (Figure 8.1).
- Tilted patient position is replaced by lateral uterine displacement (LUD) (Figure 8.2). LUD displaces the uterus to the left in order to alleviate aortocaval compression (may occur at 20 weeks of gestational age or earlier). In the case of one rescuer, LUD is not feasible and therefore the patient should be placed, if at all possible, in tilted position as per the old recommendations. In a two-rescuer situation, one of the rescuers applies LUD while the other completes the compression/ventilation cycles. The rescuers switch roles every 2 minutes.
- Rate, depth of compressions, and compression/ventilation ratio remain unchanged.

Box 8.1 Causes of cardiac arrest during pregnancy.

Nonobstetric

- Anaphylaxis
- Anesthetic complications
- Aortic dissection
- Bleeding (splenic artery rupture, hepatic rupture, disseminated intravascular coagulation)
- Cardiac causes (arrhythmias, myocardial infarction)
- Drugs (magnesium sulfate, local anesthetic toxicity, illicit drugs)
- Hypoglycemia
- Pulmonary embolism
- Sepsis
- Stroke
- Trauma

Obstetric

- Amniotic fluid embolism
- Bleeding (uterine atony, placental abruption, placenta previa)
- Eclampsia
- Gestational hypertension
- HELLP syndrome (hemolysis, elevated liver enzymes, low platelet count)
- Idiopathic peripartum cardiomyopathy
- Preeclampsia

Early warning signs

- Changes in blood pressure, heart rate, respiratory rate, oxygen saturation
- Oliguria
- Signs of maternal cognitive dysfunction
- End organ dysfunction

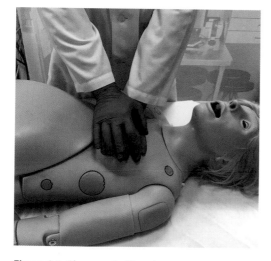

Figure 8.1 Placement of hands.

- An AED, if available, should be used without hesitation. There is no evidence to suggest that the use of biphasic truncated waveform defibrillation can affect the heart of the fetus. If the patient recovers, she should be placed in the lateral decubitus position to avoid aortocaval compression.

ACLS

When early warning signs are present and the patient becomes unstable. the following actions should be taken to prevent the condition progressing to cardiac arrest.

- The patient should be placed in a full left lateral decubitus position to relieve aortocaval compression.
- Administration of 100% oxygen by face mask to treat or prevent hypoxemia is recommended.
- Intravenous access should be established above the diaphragm to ensure that intravenously administered therapy is not obstructed by the gravid uterus.
- Precipitating factors should be investigated and treated.

In-hospital cardiac arrest response in pregnancy is an event requiring the collaboration of three teams:

- regular code response team
- obstetric team
- neonatal resuscitation team.

(a)

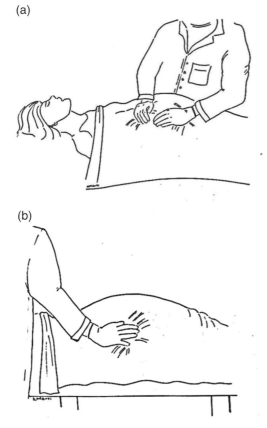

(b)

Figure 8.2 (a) LUD from the patient's left side. (b) LUD from the patient's right side.

ACLS is performed similarly to adult resuscitation; certain issues warrant consideration due to changes in the anatomy and physiology of the pregnant patient. Airway management is more challenging in pregnancy due to significant upper airway mucosal changes (friability, edema) and gastric hypokinesis, leading to a potentially higher risk of gastric content aspiration. Oxygen requirements are higher for the pregnant patient and therefore ventilation and oxygenation are also more challenging.

Defibrillation and doses of medication used in resuscitation are the same as those required for adults with cardiac arrest.

A pharmacologic consideration unique to maternal cardiac arrest is the potential utilization of lipid emulsion therapy. This is indicated in cases of in-hospital maternal cardiac arrest resulting from local anesthetic toxicity. The risks of administering "lipid rescue" appear to be minimal and may be life-saving in the obstetric patient. If local anesthetic toxicity has resulted in refractory maternal cardiac arrest, extracorporeal membrane oxygenation (ECMO) or cardiopulmonary bypass should be considered.

Changes in the standard ACLS protocol that have been recommended in the management of maternal cardiac arrest include the following.

• Application of cricoid pressure in obstetric patients to reduce the risk of aspiration is not justified because of paucity of data.
• Postshock rhythm evaluation is no longer endorsed by the AHA, so that interruptions in high-quality CPR are minimized.
• Vasopressin is no longer recommended as an alternative to epinephrine during ACLS in the pregnant patient, given its potential effects on the uterus.

Perimortem Cesarean Delivery

ACLS guidelines recommend that "if the mother's pulse has not been restored within 4–5 minutes, perimortem cesarean delivery should be performed. Fetal viability must be considered in this decision."

Although it is sometimes difficult to estimate date of pregnancy, there are some accepted "rule of thumb" landmarks. Gestational age is 12 weeks if the uterus is palpable above the pubic symphysis, 20 weeks if the uterus is palpable at the level of the umbilicus, 24–36 weeks if the uterus is palpable at the level of the xiphoid process. In case of a previable past-20 weeks pregnancy, perimortem delivery is also shown to have maternal benefit. Even in cases of a delayed birth – past 5 minutes of resuscitative effort – and for a patient with a viable gestation, the uterus needs to be evacuated to maximize maternal survival.

Note: It seems that ACLS courses do not routinely address the pregnant patient population. Good planning and scenario-based simulations may help to improve outcomes and team response in the event of cardiac arrest during pregnancy.

Further Reading

Aloizos S, Seretis C, Liakos N, *et al.* (2013) HELLP syndrome: understanding and management of a pregnancy-specific disease. *Journal of Obstetrics and Gynecology*, **33**, 331.

Balki M, Liu S, León JA, *et al.* (2017) Epidemiology of cardiac arrest during hospitalization for delivery in Canada: a nationwide study. *Anesthesia and Analgesia*, **124**, 890.

Briller J. (2016) Cardiac arrest in pregnancy: 10 things to know. Available online at: http://2016.cppcongress.com/wp-content/uploads/2016/03/Cardiac-Arrest-Top10-Things-to-Know.pdf (accessed 15 October 2017).

Cambel T and Sanson T. (2009) Cardiac arrest and pregnancy. *Journal of Emergencies, Trauma and Shock*, **2**, 34.

Cobb B and Lipman S. (2017) Cardiac arrest: obstetric CPR/ACLS. *Clinical Obstetrics and Gynecology*, **60**, 425.

European Resuscitation Council (2000) Part 8: Advanced Challenges in Resuscitation. Section 3: Special Challenges in ECC. 3 F: Cardiac Arrest Associated with Pregnancy. European Resuscitation Council. *Resuscitation*, **46**, 293.

Jeejeebhoy FM, Zelop CM, Lipman S, *et al.* (2015) Cardiac arrest in pregnancy: a scientific statement from the American Heart Association. *Circulation*, **132**, 1747.

Killion M. (2015) Cardiac arrest in pregnancy. *MCN: American Journal of Maternal/Child Nursing*, **40**, 262.

Lipman S, Cohen S, and Einav S. (2014) The Society for Obstetric Anesthesia and Perinatology consensus statement on the management of cardiac arrest in pregnancy. *Anesthesia and Analgesia*, **118**, 1003.

Mallampalli A and Guy E. (2005) Cardiac arrest in pregnancy and somatic support after brain death. *Critical Care Medicine*, **33**, S325.

Mauer DK, Gervais HW, Dick WF, *et al.* (1993) Cardiopulmonary resuscitation (CPR) during pregnancy: Working Group on CPR of the European Academy of Anaesthesiology. *European Journal of Anaesthesiology*, **10**, 437.

Morris S and Stacey M. (2003) Resuscitation in pregnancy. *British Medical Journal*, **327**, 1277.

Peters CW, Layon AJ, and Edwards RK. (2005) Cardiac arrest during pregnancy. *Journal of Clinical Anesthesia*, **17**, 229.

Rees GAD and Willis BA. (1998) Resuscitation in late pregnancy. *Anesthesia*, **43**, 347.

Sogut O, Kamaz A, and Erdogan MO. (2010) Successful cardiopulmonary resuscitation in pregnancy: a case report. *Journal of Clinical Medicine Research*, **2**, 50.

Vanden Hoek TL, Morrison LJ, Shuster, M, *et al.* (2010) Part 12: Cardiac Arrest in Special Situations: 2010 American Heart Association Guidelines for Cardiopulmonary Resuscitation and Emergency Cardiovascular Care. *Circulation*, **122**, S829.

Whitty JE. (2002) Maternal cardiac arrest in pregnancy. *Clinical Obstetrics and Gynecology*, **45**, 377.

9

Obstetric-Gynecologic Emergencies

Christos A. Skouteris

Gynecologic emergencies are disease conditions of the female reproductive system that threaten the life of the woman, her sexual function, and the perpetuation of her fertility. Common gynecologic emergencies present as acute abdomen, abnormal vaginal bleeding, or a combination of both, and are often related to early pregnancy complications, pelvic inflammatory disease (PID), and contraceptive issues.

The basic objective of this chapter is two-fold: to provide an overview of these emergency gynecologic conditions on an individual basis and to discuss the actions that should be taken if these gynecologic emergency conditions develop when the pregnant patient is under the care of the dental practitioner. Time is of the essence in these cases and so often there is an overlap in the management steps, with some requiring immediate resuscitation.

The following obstetric-gynecologic conditions that can escalate to true emergency situations will be discussed in this chapter:

- Hypertensive disorders of pregnancy
- Abdominal pain in pregnancy
- Vaginal bleeding in pregnancy
- Labor and on-scene delivery.

Hypertensive Disorders of Pregnancy

There are four categories of hypertension in pregnancy:

- preeclampsia and eclampsia
- chronic hypertension (of any cause, that predates pregnancy)
- chronic hypertension with superimposed preeclampsia
- gestational hypertension (blood pressure elevation after 20 weeks of gestation in the absence of proteinuria, thrombocytopenia, elevated LFTs, renal insufficiency, pulmonary edema, or new-onset cerebral or visual disturbances).

Discussion in this chapter will focus only on preeclampsia and eclampsia (Box 9.1).

Preeclampsia

Preeclampsia is defined as hypertension in association with thrombocytopenia (platelet count less than 100 000/mL), impaired liver function (elevated blood levels of liver transaminases to twice the normal concentration), the new development of renal insufficiency (elevated serum creatinine greater

Dental Management of the Pregnant Patient, First Edition. Edited by Christos A. Skouteris.
© 2018 John Wiley & Sons, Inc. Published 2018 by John Wiley & Sons, Inc.

Box 9.1 Complications of severe preeclampsia and eclampsia.

Maternal	Fetal
Pulmonary edema	Oligohydramnios
Oliguria and acute renal failure	Intrauterine growth restriction
Subcapsular hepatic hemorrhage with right upper quadrant pain	Absent or reverse end-diastolic flow in the umbilical artery
	Preterm birth
Liver rupture	Fetal demise
Placental abruption	
Blurred vision	
Photophobia	
Loss of vision	
Hyperreflexia	
HELLP syndrome (HEmolysis, elevated Liver enzymes, and Low Platelet count)	
Stroke	

---

than 1.1 mg/dL), pulmonary edema, or new-onset cerebral or visual disturbances. Under the new ACOG guidelines, dependence of the diagnosis of preeclampsia on the presence of proteinuria has been eliminated.

Symptoms and Signs

Mild Preeclampsia
- Hypertension (blood pressure greater than or equal to 140 mmHg systolic or greater than or equal to 90 mmHg diastolic on two occasions 4 hours apart after 20 weeks of gestation in a woman with previously normal blood pressure)
- Peripheral edema (from water retention)

Severe Preeclampsia
- Hypertension (systolic blood pressure 160 mmHg or higher, or diastolic blood pressure 100 mmHg or higher on two occasions at least 4 hours apart when the patient is resting)

- Headache
- Visual changes
- Shortness of breath
- Chest pain
- Epigastric or right upper quadrant pain
- Persistent nausea/vomiting

Cause

Unknown. Recent studies indicate the possible implication of abnormal placental perfusion and syncytiotrophoblast (STB) stress in the development of early and late preeclampsia.

Maternal Risk Factors
- Extremes of age
- First pregnancy
- New paternity
- Multiparity
- *In vitro* fertilization
- Obesity
- Personal or family history of preeclampsia
- Smoking
- Diabetes mellitus
- Preexisting hypertension
- Renal disease

Action

Elevated blood pressure to the level of *mild preeclampsia* +/- evidence of peripheral edema, in a previously normotensive pregnant patient.

- Consider preexisting hypertension (from medical Hx).
- Consider dental anxiety.
- Consider preeclampsia risk factors.
- Defer treatment and contact/refer to obstetrician-gynecologist.

Elevated blood pressure to the level of *severe preeclampsia* plus one or more of the signs and symptoms mentioned earlier.

- Activate EMS for immediate transport: life-threatening emergency.
- Monitor vital signs.
- Notify patient's obstetrician-gynecologist as soon as possible.

Eclampsia

Eclampsia is diagnosed when preeclampsia is accompanied by generalized seizures. Most often, it develops in the context of severe preeclampsia, but sometimes occurs when the disease has been mild.

Symptoms and Signs
The signs and symptoms of severe preeclampsia plus seizures.

Cause and Risk Factors
As for eclampsia.

Action
Elevated blood pressure plus one or more of the signs and symptoms of severe preeclampsia plus seizures.

- Activate EMS for immediate transport: life-threatening emergency.
- Monitor vital signs.
- Protect patient during seizure activity.
- Notify patient's obstetrician-gynecologist as soon as possible.

Abdominal Pain in Pregnancy

Abdominal pain is the most frequent complaint during pregnancy. Although often it may be related to anatomic, physiologic, biochemical, and positional changes during pregnancy, it is essential to rule out "pathologic" obstetric and nonobstetric causes. Nonobstetric causes are the same as those triggering abdominal pain in the general population (e.g., appendicitis, peptic ulcer disease, etc.). There are also nonobstetric causes of abdominal pain that are associated with pregnancy (e.g., acute fatty liver, acute cholecystitis). Discussion of the nonobstetric causes of abdominal pain in pregnancy is beyond the scope of this chapter. Reference will focus on the obstetric causes of abdominal pain (Box 9.2).

Box 9.2 Abdominal pain in pregnancy: obstetric-gynecologic causes.

Early pregnancy	Late pregnancy
Spontaneous abortion	Preterm labor
Ectopic pregnancy	Placental abruption
Ovarian hyperstimulation syndrome	Uterine rupture
Ovarian cyst/Ovarian torsion	Chorioamnionitis
Fibroid torsion/degeneration	Acute polyhydramnios
	Preeclampsia/HELLP syndrome

Abdominal Pain in Early Pregnancy

Spontaneous Abortion
Symptoms and Signs This is the most common cause of bleeding in the first half of pregnancy, with more than 80% occurring in the first 12 weeks. Signs and symptoms of spontaneous abortion are abdominal, pelvic, or back pain usually accompanied by light bleeding (spotting), frank vaginal bleeding, and visualization of products of conception (blood clots and tissue).

Action
- Activate EMS for immediate transport.
- Monitor vital signs.
- Sterile towel over vagina.
- Replace and save blood-soaked towels.
- Save all tissue. Blood-soaked towels and tissues should accompany patient during transfer.
- Notify patient's obstetrician-gynecologist as soon as possible.

Ectopic Pregnancy
Symptoms and Signs
Ectopic pregnancy is defined as the presence of a pregnancy outside the uterine cavity (most commonly in the fallopian tubes; Figure 9.1). It may present with subtle symptoms

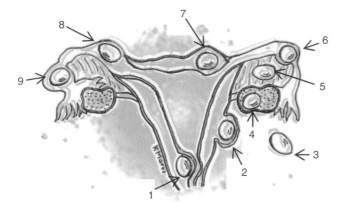

Figure 9.1 Sites of ectopic fertilized ovum implantation. 1. Cervical, 2. Intramural, 3. Abdominal, 4. Ovarian, 5. Interligamentous, 6. Ampullar tubal, 7. Interstitial, 8. Isthmic tubal, 9. Infundibular fimbrial.

such as mild abdominal pain, typically unilateral, associated with vaginal spotting or as an acute event in cases of a ruptured ectopic pregnancy (sharp, stabbing abdominal pain and varying degrees of hemodynamic instability, ranging from changes in pulse rate or blood pressure to maternal collapse).

Ectopic pregnancy is responsible for a considerable proportion of maternal mortality and morbidity. According to the WHO, ectopic pregnancy accounts for 0.1–4.9% of the total maternal deaths worldwide. Ruptured ectopic pregnancy is a true medical emergency. The rule of thumb is that *sudden acute abdominal pain in early pregnancy should be considered as ruptured ectopic pregnancy until proven otherwise.*

Action
- Activate EMS for immediate transportation.
- Monitor vital signs.
- Apply BLS if maternal collapse (see Chapter 8).
- Notify patient's obstetrician-gynecologist as soon as possible.

Ovarian Hyperstimulation Syndrome
Symptoms and Signs Symptoms include acute abdominal pain, rapid abdominal distension (secondary to ascites), headache, vomiting and in some cases oliguria. Severe cases can be life-threatening and for these cases, admission to hospital is required.

Action
- Activate EMS for immediate transportation.
- Monitor vital signs.
- Apply BLS if needed (see Chapter 8).
- Notify patient's obstetrician-gynecologist as soon as possible.

Ovarian Cyst/Ovarian Torsion
Symptoms and Signs Intermittent and unilateral abdominal pain, nausea, vomiting, and general malaise.

Action
- Activate EMS for immediate transportation.
- Notify patient's obstetrician-gynecologist as soon as possible.

Fibroid Torsion/Degeneration
Symptoms and Signs Severe localized abdominal pain, nausea and vomiting.

Action
- Activate EMS for immediate transportation.
- Notify patient's obstetrician-gynecologist as soon as possible.

Abdominal Pain in Late Pregnancy

Preterm Labor
Symptoms and Signs Preterm labor often presents with intermittent abdominal pain and uterine contractions, preceded or not by preterm rupture of membranes.

Action
- Activate EMS for immediate transportation.
- Prepare for on-scene delivery (see Labor and on-scene delivery later in the chapter).
- Notify patient's obstetrician-gynecologist as soon as possible.

Placental Abruption

Placental abruption is defined as premature separation of a normally inserted placenta (Figure 9.2).

Symptoms and Signs The classic symptoms are acute and severe abdominal pain, sustained uterine contraction, Couvelaire uterus (secondary to the presence of blood into the myometrium), +/−vaginal bleeding. In severe cases, the patient can present with signs of hypovolemic shock.

Action
- Activate EMS for immediate transportation.
- Monitor vital signs.
- Apply BLS if needed (see Chapter 8).
- Notify patient's obstetrician-gynecologist as soon as possible.

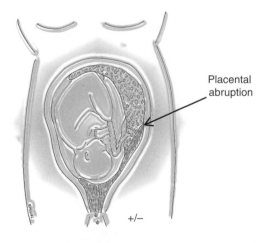

Placental abruption

+/−

Figure 9.2 Placental abruption may or may not be associated with vaginal bleeding.

Chorioamnionitis

The presence of chorioamnionitis is typically associated with a history of prolonged rupture of membranes, but it can also happen with intact amniotic membranes.

Symptoms and Signs Abdominal pain associated with systemic symptoms and signs of infection such as maternal tachycardia, pyrexia, and offensive vaginal discharge. Unlikely to develop as an acute event during dental care.

Action
- Activate EMS for immediate transportation.
- Monitor vital signs.
- Notify patient's obstetrician-gynecologist as soon as possible.

Acute Polyhydramnios

A sudden increase in amniotic fluid causes uterine distension and the patient presents with a tense abdomen causing breathlessness.

Action
- Activate EMS for immediate transportation.
- Monitor vital signs.
- Notify patient's obstetrician-gynecologist as soon as possible.

HELLP Syndrome (HEmolysis, Elevated Liver enzymes and Low Platelets)

Symptoms and Signs The patient may present with severe epigastric and right upper quadrant pain secondary to edema of the liver capsule. Other classic symptoms of preeclampsia include headache, visual disturbances, nausea and vomiting, irritability, and altered consciousness.

Action
- Activate EMS for immediate transportation.
- Monitor vital signs.
- Apply BLS if altered consciousness.
- Notify patient's obstetrician-gynecologist as soon as possible.

Vaginal Bleeding in Pregnancy

Vaginal Bleeding in the First Half of Pregnancy

Twenty to thirty percent of women experience vaginal bleeding in the first half of pregnancy. Box 9.3 lists the main causes of vaginal bleeding in early and late pregnancy.

- *Implantation bleeding*: during implantation, many women may experience implantation bleeding as the trophoblastic tissue embeds into the myometrium. This bleeding is characteristically light, occurs earlier than expected, and is of shorter duration than a normal menstrual period.
- *Spontaneous abortion.*
- *Anembryonic pregnancy*: anembryonic pregnancy, previously termed "blighted ovum," is a nonviable intrauterine pregnancy. Presentation is indistinguishable from other causes of bleeding in early pregnancy.
- *Ectopic pregnancy.*
- *Gestational trophoblastic disease*: gestational trophoblastic disease (GTD) is a group of benign and malignant tumors that arise from trophoblastic cells of the placenta. These tumors secrete high levels of beta-hCG and therefore cause symptoms similar to early pregnancy. The most common clinical manifestation is vaginal bleeding.

Vaginal Bleeding in the Second Half of Pregnancy

- *Placenta previa*: in placenta previa, the placenta implants in the lower uterine segment, near or covering, the internal cervical os (Figure 9.3). Placenta previa is thought to be responsible for about 5% of all miscarriages. It frequently causes very light bleeding (spotting) early in pregnancy. Occasionally, after 28 weeks of pregnancy placenta previa can cause episodes of significant bleeding. Usually, the bleeding occurs suddenly and is bright red. The bleeding is rarely accompanied with pain and it usually stops by itself. About 25% of such patients will go into labor within the next several days. Sometimes, placenta previa does not cause bleeding until labor has already begun.
- *Placental abruption.*
- *Vasa previa*: under normal circumstances, the fetal vessels are housed in the umbilical cord, which inserts into the placenta. Under rare conditions, the fetal vessels run through the fetal membranes without the protection of the cord and cross the internal os before they reach the placenta. Because they lie between the fetus and the cervix, there is no way to prevent trauma to these vessels when the membranes rupture or childbirth occurs.
- *Uterine rupture*: uterine rupture is caused by a complete tear in the uterine wall and is

Box 9.3 Vaginal bleeding in pregnancy.

Early pregnancy	Late pregnancy
Implantation bleeding	Placenta previa
Spontaneous abortion	Placental abruption
Anembryonic pregnancy	Vasa previa
Ectopic pregnancy	Uterine rupture
Gestational trophoblastic disease	

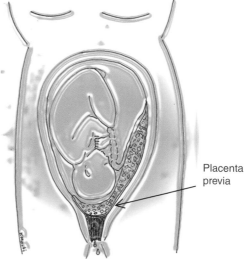

Placenta previa

Figure 9.3 The placenta is covering the cervical os.

usually associated with labor. In rare instances, it occurs spontaneously in the second half of pregnancy. Symptoms of uterine rupture not associated with labor can be misleading. Abdominal pain and vaginal bleeding are often minimal or even absent. In extreme situations, pain and bleeding may be severe, and hypovolemic shock may ensue. The fetus may protrude into the abdominal cavity, allowing fetal parts to be palpable on abdominal exam.

Action

Any episode of vaginal bleeding in pregnancy when the patient is in the dental office should be considered an emergency and prompt appropriate action should be taken.

- EMS activation for immediate transportation.
- Monitoring of vital signs.
- Application of BLS if needed.
- Notification of the patient's obstetrician-gynecologist as soon as possible.

Labor and On-Scene Delivery

There have been no reported incidents of a pregnant patient going into labor and delivering while undergoing dental care. However, there are numerous reports of babies having been born in the most unusual places such as in planes, taxis, on cruise ships, and even on a sidewalk in New York City in 2014. The delivery of the newborn was assisted in most occasions by people without any proper training or experience in dealing with such an occurrence. Therefore, the possibility of a patient going into labor while receiving dental care should not be regarded as an event that can never occur.

The purpose of discussing the issue of labor and on-scene delivery is to provide some practical information that would be helpful to the dental practitioner should the need arise. It is highly recommended that the practitioner utilize the high-fidelity simulation that is available for familiarization with procedures and management of clinical situations, emergency or otherwise. Instructional videos and high-fidelity simulation offered by academic and other institutional simulation centers provide excellent information and hands-on training on normal spontaneous vaginal delivery.

With the understanding that readers might already have personal or professional experience on the subject, a pictorial presentation of simulated normal spontaneous delivery is included in this chapter. The discussion of fetal dystocia, with presentations such as breech (frank, complete, single or double footling), occiput posterior, face or brow, transverse lie, and shoulder dystocia is beyond the scope of this book. Fetal dystocia may occur when the fetus is too large for the pelvic opening (fetopelvic disproportion) or is abnormally positioned (e.g., breech presentation). Normal fetal presentation is vertex, with the occiput anterior. Excellent reference on these topics enriched by high-quality video presentations can be found in the obstetrics and gynecology online professional version of the Merck Manual (www.merckmanuals.com/professional/gynecology-and-obstetrics).

Stages of Labor

There are three stages of labor.

First Stage
The first stage – from onset of labor to full dilation of the cervix (about 10 cm) – has two phases, latent and active. Pushing or bearing down is not effective during this stage and is harmful in that it may cause a tearing of the cervix.

Latent Phase
- Longest stage.
- Progressive coordination of irregular contractions.
- Thinning of the cervix (effacement).
- Cervix dilates from 4 to 6 cm.
- Bloody show before or during this stage.

- Amniotic sac may break before or during this stage.
- For a first child, this stage can average 18 hours or more.

Active Phase

- Full cervical dilation at 10 cm.
- The leading anatomical part of the fetus (presenting part) descends into the midpelvis.
- Amniotomy (if the membranes have not ruptured spontaneously).

Second Stage

The second stage is the time from full cervical dilation to delivery of the fetus.

- Baby enters birth canal.
- Ferguson's reflex: urge to push as baby's body puts pressure on the perineum.
- Crowning (presenting part appears at the vaginal opening):
  - cephalic presentation – head first
  - breech presentation – buttocks or both feet first.

Third Stage

The third stage of labor begins after delivery of the infant and ends with delivery of the placenta. This stage usually takes only a few minutes but may last up to 30 minutes.

False Labor: Braxton Hicks Contractions

Braxton Hicks contractions ("false" labor pain) occur in the third trimester but also as early as the second trimester and are due to occasional tightening and relaxing of the uterus. Box 9.4 summarizes the differences between Braxton Hicks contractions and labor contractions.

On-Scene Delivery

> "It always seems impossible until it is done." (Nelson Mandela)

A spontaneous normal delivery can occur as a prehospital event. Under certain circumstances, it can develop into an "emergency situation" requiring prompt action. Therefore, a on-scene delivery may be inevitable. Circumstances that could lead to the need for a on-scene delivery include:

- no suitable transportation
- adverse weather conditions
- distance to hospital
- hospital or physician can't be reached
- delivery is imminent (contractions less than 2 minutes apart).

If a on-scene delivery is to occur in the dental office, the following actions should be performed.

Box 9.4 Braxton Hicks contractions vs labor contractions.	
Braxton Hicks contractions	**Labor contractions**
Infrequent in nature, occur every 5–10 minutes a few times a day	Occur more regularly, usually 2 to 3 minutes apart
Not constant, do not last longer than a few seconds	Each one tends to last for 30 to 90 seconds
Severity depends on activity level and position	Remain consistent regardless of activity level and position
Usually quite weak or strong in the beginning, weaker with time	Cause a sharp pain
Felt primarily in the lower abdomen (sometimes in the upper abdomen)	May begin in the abdomen moving toward the lower back or vice versa

Source: Adapted from: What are False Contractions? Available online at: www.pregmed.org/what-are-false-contractions. htm (accessed 24 October 2017).

Identify That the Patient is Going into Labor

- Crowning has occurred.
- Contractions closer than 2 minutes apart, intense, last 30–90 seconds.
- Patient has the urge to push.
- Patient's abdomen is hard.
- Activate EMS.
- If birth does not occur within 10 minutes, transport patient.

Prepare for Delivery

- Stay calm and prepare for delivery.
- Explain to the patient that the infant will need to be delivered in the office.
- Calm and reassure the patient, protect her privacy.
- Don't allow the patient to use the bathroom.

- Ensure mother's comfort.
- Position patient on the dental chair on her back with the legs apart, flexed at the knees and resting on two stools or chairs. Keep the footrest of the dental chair down.
- Apply body substance isolation (BSI) precautions (gown, mask, gloves).
- Apply sterile towels under the buttocks and around the vaginal opening.
- Do not touch the vaginal area except to deliver and in the presence of your assistant.

Delivery
Points to Note

- If the amniotic sack is not broken, a finger is used to rupture the sack and drain the amniotic fluid. Note the color and consistency of the fluid.

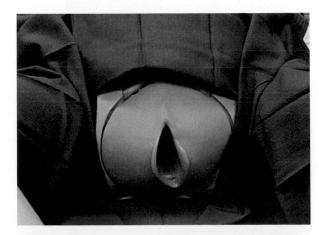

Figure 9.4 Ask the patient to bear down (push) and look for bulging of the perineum. The hand could be inserted through the vaginal opening at this point to make sure that a normal vertex presentation is in progress by feeling for fetal sutures and fontanelles.

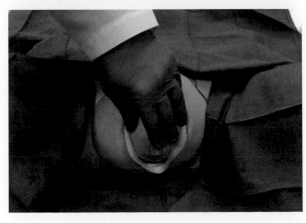

Figure 9.5 Encourage the mother to take a breath between contractions and to push with contractions. During crowning, apply gentle pressure against the head so that the fetal head can clear the pubic symphysis.

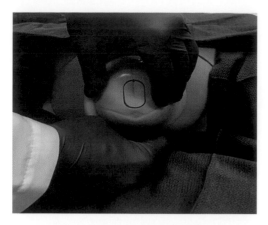

Figure 9.6 A hand is placed on the perineum and upward pressure is applied, while counterpressure on the fetal head is applied with the other hand to control head extension.

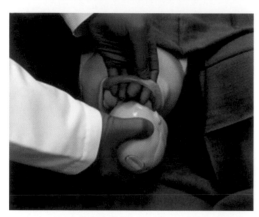

Figure 9.7 Identify if the nuchal cord is around the fetal neck. If so, pull the cord out and over the fetal head.

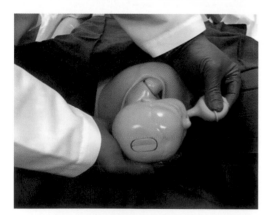

Figure 9.8 Normally the fetal head rotates spontaneously after it has fully emerged through the vaginal opening. At this time the nose and mouth of the fetus can be suctioned out. However, do not delay delivery to perform this task.

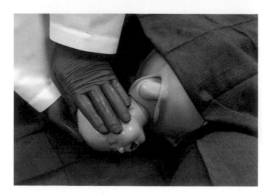

Figure 9.9 Both hands are placed on the mandible and a downward pull is applied to deliver the anterior shoulder.

Figure 9.10 Upward pull is applied to deliver the posterior shoulder.

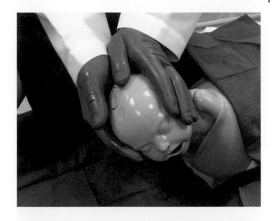

Figure 9.11 The head and torso are supported as the fetus continues to emerge through the vaginal opening.

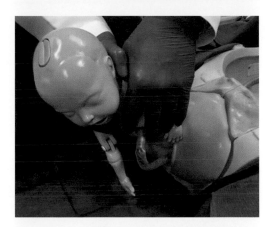

Figure 9.12 With continuous support of the head and torso, the lower extremities are delivered.

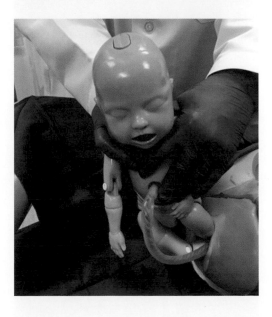

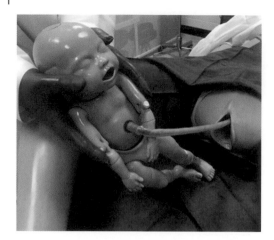

Figure 9.13 Usually, the body delivers spontaneously after the posterior shoulder. Stimulate the baby to breathe by tapping the feet, if necessary.

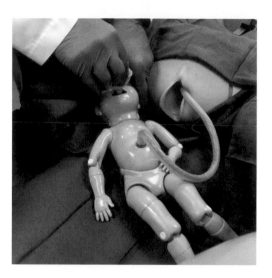

Figure 9.14 Place the baby level with the vagina and while waiting for the nuchal cord pulsations to stop before the cord is clamped and divided, suction out the mouth and nose.

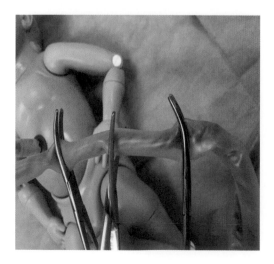

Figure 9.15 After the nuchal cord pulsations have stopped, a clamp is applied 4–5 cm from the umbilicus. Before placing the second clamp distal to the first, blood is milked out of the cord in the direction of the placenta. The second clamp is then placed and the cord is divided between clamps.

Figure 9.16 Delivery of the placenta. The cord is clamped as close to the vagina as possible. A hand is placed above the pubic symphysis and pressure is applied on the abdominal wall towards the spine. Steady, gentle pull is applied on the cord, initially in a downward direction. As more cord appears, it is reclamped close to the vagina and the pull on the cord is continuous until the placenta emerges. The placenta is then grasped with both hands, rotated, and delivered.

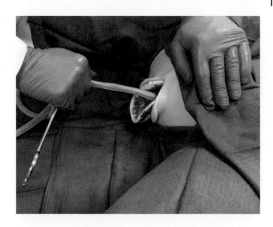

- During delivery of the head, hand pressure on the perineum also protects it from potential tear.
- If the nuchal cord cannot easily be pulled from around the fetal neck, it should be clamped and divided.
- Aggressive pulling on the fetus in an effort to deliver it as fast as possible should *absolutely be avoided.*
- Care should be exercised in handling the neonate during delivery because neonates are slippery. It is prudent to bring the footrest of the dental chair up as soon as the neonate is delivered.
- Stimulate the baby by rubbing the head and abdomen.
- If the child starts breathing and moving and appears to be in good health, turn the baby over to your assistant. Make sure that the baby is vigorously dried, suctioned, and kept warm.
- Do not stimulate the baby to cry if the birth is complicated by thick meconium (fetal feces – the amniotic fluid is thick and pea green), to avoid aspiration of fecal material.
- Do not delay transport of the mother and baby to hospital to deliver the placenta. The placenta may take up to 30 minutes to be delivered. If the placenta was delivered, it must be sent to the hospital together with the mother and newborn.
- After delivery, contraction of the myometrium is the primary means of controlling uterine bleeding. Massaging the uterine fundus by pushing gently on the mother's suprapubic abdominal wall promotes uterine contraction and hemorrhage control.
- If time and circumstances allow, calculate the Apgar score which is a measure of the physical condition of the newborn (Table 9.1).

The purpose of the information provided in this section is to present the basics of normal prehospital, spontaneous on-scene delivery. The reader is advised to review related topics available in the literature and in online media

Table 9.1 Apgar score.

	Apgar score 0	Apgar score 1	Apgar score 2
Appearance	Blue or pale all over	Extremities blue, body pink	Pink all over
Pulse rate (PR)	Absent	PR <100/min	PR >100/min
Grimace	No response to stimulation	Some response to stimulation	Crying
Activity	None	Arms and legs flexed	Active movement
Respiration	Absent	Slow and irregular	Robust cry

or to seek hands-on training in simulation centers.

The simulated normal spontaneous vaginal delivery depicted in this section was performed at the University of Michigan Clinical Simulation Center, Department of Learning Health Sciences, Michigan Medicine, Ann Arbor, Michigan.

Further Reading

Abam DS. (2015) Overview of gynaecological emergencies, in *Contemporary Gynecologic Practice*, InTech, Croatia.

Almeida Jr OD. (2011) Fimbrial ectopic pregnancy following tubal anastomosis. *Journal of the Society of Laparoendoscopic Surgeons*, **15**, 539.

American College of Obstetricians and Gynecologists, Task Force on Hypertension in Pregnancy (2013) *Hypertension in Pregnancy*. Available online at www.acog.org/Resources-And-Publications/Task-Force-and-Work-Group-Reports/Hypertension-in-Pregnancy (accessed 24 October 2017).

American College of Obstetricians and Gynecologists (2014) Committee Opinion No. 590. Preparing for Clinical Emergencies in Obstetrics and Gynecology. *Obstetrics and Gynecology*, **123**, 722.

American College of Obstetricians and Gynecologists (2015) Committee Opinion No. 644. The Apgar Score. *Obstetrics and Gynecology*, **126**, e52.

Arsove P and Krause RS. (2010) Vaginal bleeding in pregnancy: Part I. *Emergency Medicine Reports*, **31**, 257.

Arsove P and Krause RS. (2010) Vaginal bleeding in pregnancy: Part II. *Emergency Medicine Reports*, **31**, 269.

Avery DM. (2009) Obstetric emergencies. *American Journal of Clinical Medicine*, **6**, 1.

Benzoni TE. (2015) *Labor and Delivery in the Emergency Department*. Available online at: https://emedicine.medscape.com/article/796379-overview (accessed 24 October 2017).

Bouyer J, Coste J, Fernandez H, *et al.* (2002) Sites of ectopic pregnancy: a 10 year population-based study of 1800 cases. *Human Reproduction*, **17**, 3224.

Carson-DeWitt R. (2011) Placenta previa, in *The Gale Encyclopedia of Medicine*, vol. 5, 4th edn (ed. LJ Fundukian), Gale, Detroit, pp. 3423–3425.

Ishimine P. (2015) Vaginal bleeding in pregnancy, in *Rosen & Barkin's 5-Minute Emergency Medicine Consult*, 5th edn, Wolters Kluwer, New York, pp. 1196–1198.

Johnston RC, Stephenson ML, Paraghamian S, *et al.* (2016) Assessing progression from mild to severe preeclampsia in expectantly managed preterm parturients. *Pregnancy Hypertension*, **6**, 340.

Pinas-Carrillo A and Chandraharan E. (2017) Abdominal pain in pregnancy: a rational approach to management. *Obstetrics, Gynaecology, and Reproductive Medicine*, **27**, 4.

Rambaldi MP and Paidas MJ. (2000) Hypertensive disorders, in *Obstetric Medicine: Management of Medical Disorders in Pregnancy* (eds W Cohen and P August P), People's Medical Publishing House, Beijing, pp. 155–182.

Redman CW, Sargent IL, and Staff AC. (2014) IFPA Senior Award Lecture: Making sense of pre-eclampsia – Two placental causes of preeclampsia? *Placenta*, **35**, S20.

Tsikouras P, Dimitraki M, Ammari A, *et al.* (2011) Differential diagnosis of ectopic pregnancy - morbidity and mortality, in *Ectopic Pregnancy – Modern Diagnosis and Management* (ed. M Kamrava), InTech, Croatia, pp. 1–9.

Appendices

Appendix 1

Cardiovascular Changes

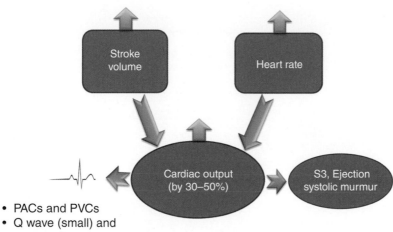

- PACs and PVCs
- Q wave (small) and inverted T wave in lead III
- ST-segment depression and T-wave inversion in the inferior and lateral leads
- Left-axis shift of QRS

Appendix 2

Cardiovascular Changes

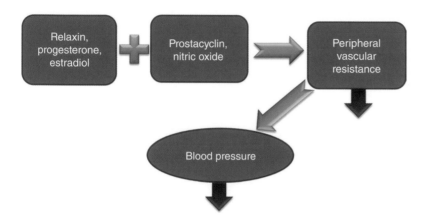

Appendix 3

Respiratory Changes

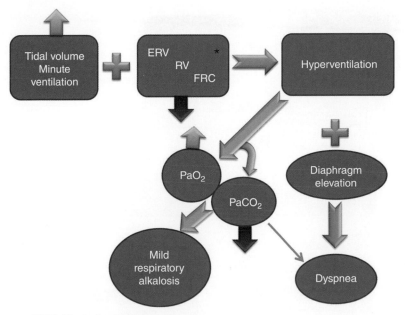

ERV: Expiratory reserve volume
RV: Residual volume
FRC: Functional residual capacity

Appendix 4

Hematologic Changes

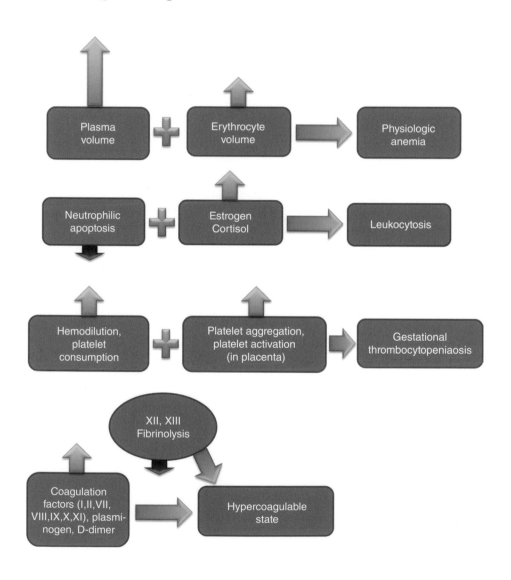

Appendix 5

Gastrointestinal Changes

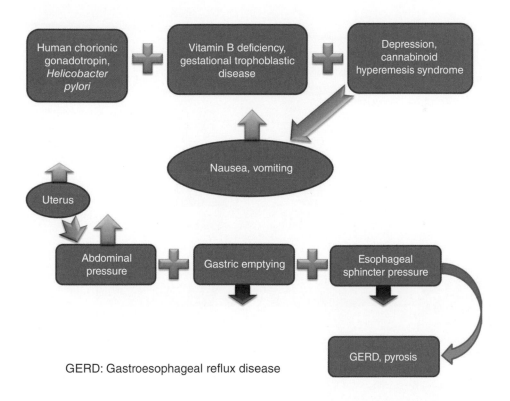

GERD: Gastroesophageal reflux disease

Appendix 6

Genitourinary Changes

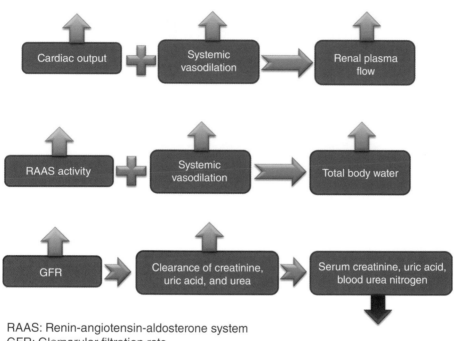

RAAS: Renin-angiotensin-aldosterone system
GFR: Glomerular filtration rate

Appendix 7

Endocrine Changes: Insulin Gestational Activity

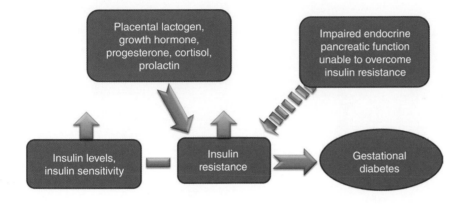

Appendix 8

OB-GYN Emergencies

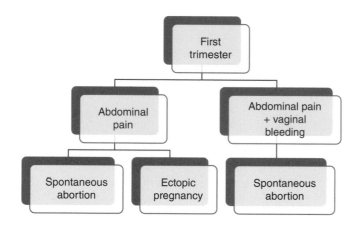

Appendix 9

OB-GYN Emergencies

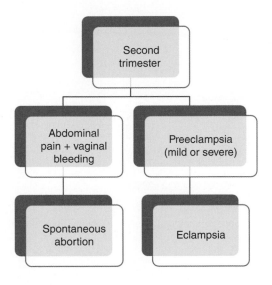

Appendix 10

OB-GYN Emergencies

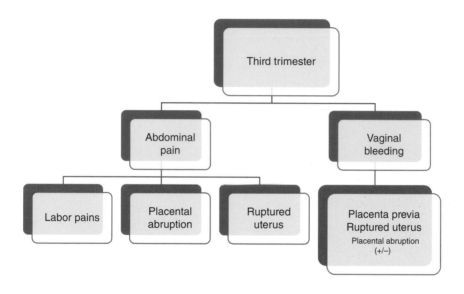

Appendix 11

Most Important Physiologic Changes Per Trimester of Pregnancy

First Trimester	Second Trimester	Third Trimester	
WEEK 1–13	WEEK 14–26	WEEK 27–40	41–42
⬇ Systemic vascular resistance (SVR)	⬇ SVR	⬇ SVR	
⬆ Cardiac output	Cardiac output ⬆	Cardiac output ⬆	
⬆ Heart rate	⬆ Heart rate	⬆ Heart rate	
⬇ Blood pressure	Blood pressure ⬇	Blood pressure ⬆	
Hyperventilation	⬆ Hyperventilation	⬆ Hyperventilation	
⬆ Dyspnea	Dyspnea ⬆	⬆ Dyspnea	
⬆ Plasma volume	⬆ Plasma volume	⬆ Plasma volume	
⬆ Physiologic anemia	Physiologic anemia ⬇	Physiologic anemia ⬆	
Hypercoagulability	Hypercoagulability	Hypercoagulability	
⬆ Leukocytosis	Leukocytosis	Leukocytosis	
⬆ Nausea/vomiting	⬇ Nausea/vomiting	Pyrosis (heartburn) ⬆	
⬆ Renal plasma flow	Renal plasma flow ⬆	⬆ Renal plasma flow	
⬆ Glomerular filtration rate (GFR)	GFR ⬆	GFR ⬆	
⬆ Aminoaciduria	⬆ Urine protein/albumin	⬆ Urine protein/albumin	
⬆ Insulin levels	Aminoaciduria ⬆	⬆ Glycosuria	
	Hydronephrosis Hydroureter	Aminoaciduria ⬆	
	⬆ Insulin levels	Hydronephrosis, hydroureter	

Appendix 12

Management of Oral Squamous Cell Carcinoma in Pregnancy

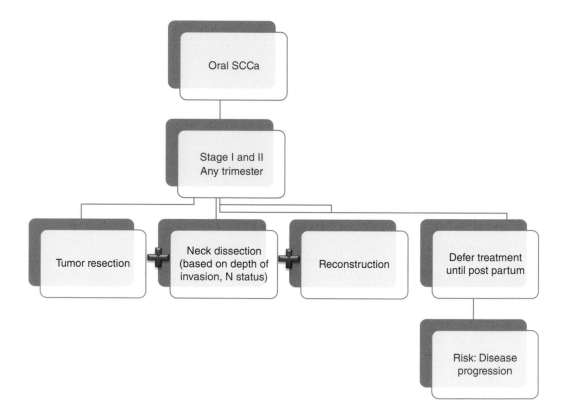

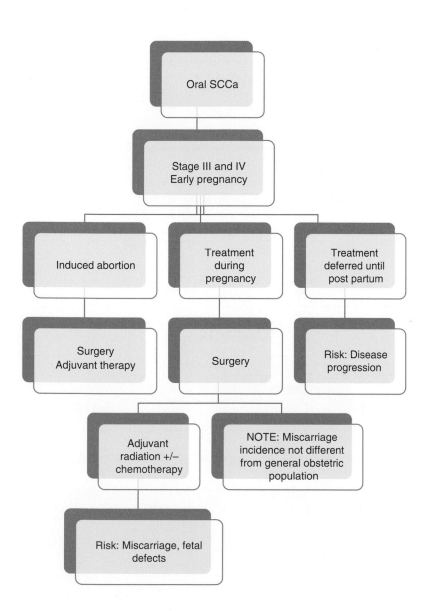

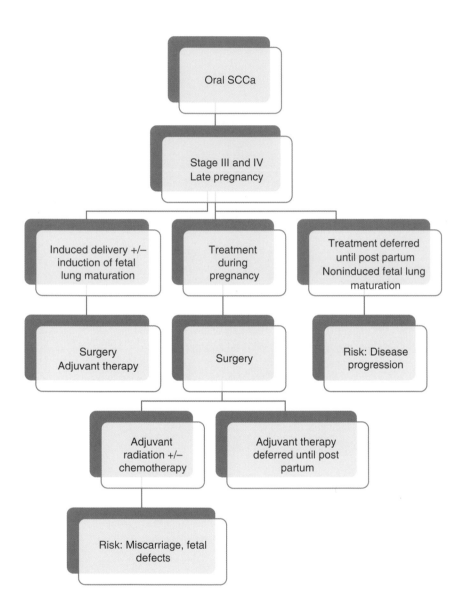

Source: Adapted from Garcia AG, Lopez JA, and Rey JMG. (2001) Squamous cell carcinoma of the maxilla during pregnancy: report of case. *Journal of Oral and Maxillofacial Surgery*, **59**, 456, with permission from Elsevier (reproduction license # 4177740725985).

Appendix 13

Management of Oral and Maxillofacial Trauma in Pregnancy

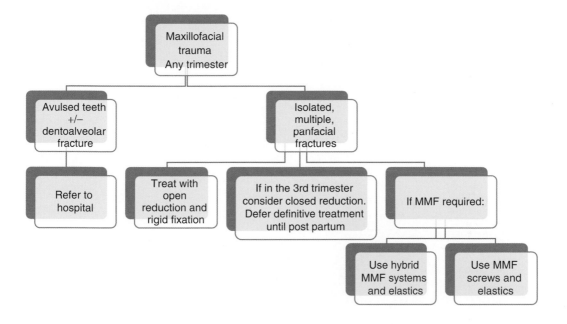

Reader's Self-Assessment Quiz

1 According to the ADA Code of Ethics, a "dentist has a duty to treat people fairly." Which of the following ethical principles is the above statement associated with?
   a Justice
   b Autonomy
   c Veracity
   d Nonmaleficence

2 Peripheral vascular resistance is more profound during:
   a the first trimester
   b labor
   c the third trimester
   d the second trimester

3 The increase in cardiac output during pregnancy:
   a is caused by an increase in stroke volume in late pregnancy
   b is caused by an increase in heart rate in early pregnancy
   c counteracts the decreased oxygen capacity of maternal blood
   d reaches its peak in the third trimester

4 The decrease in blood pressure is contributed by the action of:
   a prostacyclin
   b estradiol
   c progesterone
   d all of the above

5 Vascular remodeling in pregnancy is demonstrated by an increase in arterial compliance. A measure of increase in arterial compliance is provided by the aortic _____ index, a marker of aortic stiffness

6 Which of the following respiratory parameters remains unchanged in pregnancy?
   a Total lung volume
   b Inspiratory reserve volume
   c Expiratory reserve volume
   d Minute ventilation

7 The mild respiratory alkalosis of pregnancy is caused by:
   a an increase in arterial carbon dioxide tension
   b a decrease in arterial oxygen tension
   c a fall in serum bicarbonate
   d none of the above

8 A pregnant patient in the 34th week of gestation is found to be anemic. This condition is a result of:
   a considerable drop in red blood cell volume
   b decrease in plasma volume
   c increased red blood cell turnover
   d increase in plasma volume

9 Gestational thrombocytopenia develops from the effect of the following factors *except* for:
   a reduced platelet activation
   b hemodilution
   c increased levels of thromboxane A2
   d increased platelet aggregation

10   Pregnant women are at higher risk for thromboembolic event as a result of being in a hypercoagulable state. Which of the following coagulation factors is elevated in pregnancy?
   a   Antithrombin III
   b   Factor XII
   c   Factor XIII
   d   Factor IX

11   Hyperemesis gravidarum can cause the following conditions *except* for:
   a   emotional stress
   b   hyperthyroidism
   c   hypothyroidism
   d   vitamin B1, B6, and B12 deficiency

12   What is the percentage of pregnant women who experience pyrosis during the third trimester of pregnancy?
   a   10–25%
   b   40–85%
   c   20–30%
   d   5–15%

13   Which of the following is one of the earliest kidney functional changes that occur in pregnancy?
   a   Increase in glomerular filtration rate
   b   Increased urinary protein excretion
   c   Increased excretion of amino acids
   d   Increased excretion of glycose

14   The normal thyroid-stimulating hormone level during pregnancy is higher than the normal nonpregnancy level.
   a   True
   b   False

15   Pregnant women are at high risk for infections because they are immunosuppressed.
   a   True
   b   False

16   Vascular skin changes during pregnancy account for which of the following conditions?

   a   Dermatographism
   b   Chadwick's sign
   c   Goodell's sign
   d   All of the above

17   Which of the following is *not* a sign or symptom of supine hypotensive syndrome?
   a   Pallor
   b   Diaphoresis
   c   Bradycardia
   d   Nausea

18   From the respiratory point of view, when a pregnant patient is undergoing dental or medical treatment, the development of _____ needs to be avoided

19   The agent of choice for thromboprophylaxis in pregnancy is:
   a   unfractionated heparin
   b   coumadin
   c   low molecular weight heparin
   d   apixaban

20   A pregnant woman is susceptible to urinary tract infections because of the following conditions *except* for:
   a   glycosuria
   b   aminoaciduria
   c   increased ureteral tone
   d   asymptomatic bacteriuria

21   What percentage of pregnancies is complicated by gestational diabetes mellitus?
   a   15%
   b   7%
   c   25%
   d   10–20%

22   Pemphigoid gestationis affects only the skin and is an autoimmune subepidermal blistering disease associated with pregnancy
   a   True
   b   False

23 Which of the following statements is correct?
  a Impetigo herpetiformis is a variant of HSV
  b Oral cavity involvement is in the form of fissured tongue
  c Both are correct
  d Neither is correct

24 When a pregnant patient is sited in the dental chair, in addition to placing her in the position that prevents aortocaval compression and SHS, every effort should be made (e.g., with the use of cushions) to provide enough comfort, because close to _____% of patients experience frequent episodes of back pain

25 Pregnant women particularly during the first trimester develop an aversion to _____

26 Quantitative laboratory serum pregnancy tests detect:
  a human chorionic gonadotropin (hCG) only
  b hyperglycosylated (hCG-H) only
  c hCG and hCG-H
  d none of the above

27 Prenatal oral health counseling is very important in informing the pregnant woman on the risks that poor oral health poses for the mother and fetus. One of these risks is the vertical transmission of cariogenic *Staphylococcus aureus* from the mother to the infant with a significant risk for future caries experience and potentially low infant birth weight
  a True
  b False

28 Pregnancy gingivitis is considered the most common oral manifestation in pregnancy and reaches its peak:
  a in the second month of gestation
  b in the sixth month of gestation
  c in the eight month of gestation
  d at term

29 Which of the following is *not* part of the recommendations regarding the dental management of a patient in the first trimester of pregnancy?
  a Educate the patient about maternal oral changes during pregnancy
  b Emphasize strict oral hygiene instructions and thereby plaque control
  c Scaling, polishing, and curettage may be performed if necessary
  d Avoid routine radiographs. Use selectively and when needed

30 What measures are required if amalgam is to be used for dental restorations in pregnant women?
  i Use of rubber dam
  ii Scavenger system
  iii Avoid overfilling
  iv Polish restorations shortly after placement
  a (i) and (ii) only
  b (i), (ii), and (iii) only
  c (i), (ii), and (iv) only
  d (ii), (iii), and (iv) only

31 In composite restorations, the highest percentage of uncured monomer is present in the _____ _____ _____

32 Physiologic changes in pregnancy that may contribute to the development, severity, and complications of odontogenic infections include the following *except* for:
  a the decrease in blood pressure
  b the physiologic anemia of pregnancy
  c the gastroesophageal reflux
  d the increase in heart rate

33 Which is the most important sign or symptom that would dictate hospital referral of a pregnant patient with an odontogenic infection?
  a Fever
  b Dysphagia
  c Trismus
  d Airway compromise

34 Which of the following statements regarding the indications for removal of an epulis of pregnancy is *not* true?
   a The epulis should be removed if it is traumatized by opposing teeth resulting in pain and bleeding
   b When it interferes with normal speech and/or mastication
   c It should always be removed when it develops during pregnancy
   d When it bleeds spontaneously without prior trauma

35 Maternal physiologic changes that can influence the surgical and adjuvant treatment of malignancy in pregnancy include the following *except* for:
   a hypercoagulability
   b immunosuppression
   c hypermetabolism
   d decreased albumin levels

36 Which of the following statements relative to the expected increase in the incidence of oral cancer in pregnant women is *not* true?
   a Young females start to smoke early in life
   b An increased incidence of oral cancer is already seen in young female nonsmokers
   c Women tend to delay childbearing to an older age
   d All of the above statements are true

37 A pregnant woman in her 29th week of pregnancy presents to the dental office with partially avulsed anterior maxillary teeth secondary to domestic violence. The proper management of this patient requires:
   a splinting of the partially avulsed teeth with composite resin
   b splinting with brackets and orthodontic wire
   c hospital referral
   d referral to an oral surgery practice

38 Which of the following statements relative to the treatment of facial fractures in pregnancy is *not* true?
   a Long-term maxillomandibular fixation (MMF) is always required to ascertain fracture stability and correct occlusion in pregnant as in nonpregnant women
   b Fracture treatment could be temporized with closed reduction until post partum
   c Rigid fixation of maxillary and mandibular fractures is advisable to avoid or minimize the period of maxillomandibular fixation (MMF)
   d All of the above statements are true

39 Which of the following local anesthetics should be used with caution in a breastfeeding patient?
   a Articaine
   b Prilocaine
   c Mepivacaine
   d Bupivacaine

40 Which of the following analgesics should be used with caution during breastfeeding?
   a Ibuprofen
   b Codeine
   c Aspirin
   d Morphine

41 Metronidazole should be avoided during breastfeeding because:
   a it can alter the oral flora of the newborn
   b it gives maternal milk an unpleasant taste
   c it can reach toxic blood levels in the newborn even in recommended doses
   d all of the above

42 Which of the following corticosteroids is safe to be given to a breastfeeding mother?
   a Betamethasone
   b Prednisone
   c Dexamethasone
   d Hydrocortisone

43 Which of the following statements is *true* when performing BLS on an unconscious pregnant patient?
   a Chest compressions are performed with the patient in a 15–30° tilted position
   b Chest compressions are performed with the patient in supine position
   c Hands are placed slightly higher on the sternum
   d AED should not be used because it can affect the fetal heart

44 Which of the following conditions is less likely to cause cardiac arrest in pregnancy?
   a Amniotic fluid embolism
   b Eclampsia
   c Ectopic pregnancy
   d Anesthetic complications

45 Which of the conditions listed below differentiates severe preeclampsia from eclampsia?
   a Hypertension
   b Visual changes
   c Chest pain
   d Seizures

46 Which of the conditions that cause abdominal pain in pregnancy is considered a life-threatening emergency?
   a Placenta previa
   b Placental abruption
   c Ectopic pregnancy
   d Spontaneous abortion

47 If a spontaneous abortion occurs while a pregnant patient is under treatment in the dental office, all blood-soaked towels, blood clots, and tissues should be disposed immediately as a potential biohazard.
   a True
   b False

48 The conditions listed below can cause bleeding in late pregnancy *except* for:
   a anembryonic pregnancy
   b vasa previa

   c placental abruption
   d placenta previa

49 What are the most important actions during an ob-gyn emergency situation occurring in the dental office?
   a Activate EMS for immediate transport
   b Monitor vital signs, perform BLS if needed
   c Notify the patient's obstetrician-gynecologist
   d All of the above

50 The latent phase of the first stage of labor is characterized by the following *except* for:
   a progressive coordination of irregular contractions
   b bloody show before or during this stage
   c Braxton Hicks contractions
   d amniotic sac may break before or during this stage

51 During spontaneous normal vaginal delivery and after the head has fully emerged, which part of the infant should be delivered next?
   a Posterior shoulder
   b Anterior shoulder
   c Right upper extremity
   d Left upper extremity

52 Which of the following protective measures render dental radiography absolutely safe for the pregnant patients?
   a Rectangular collimated beams
   b Use of high-speed films
   c Lead apron and thyroid collar
   d All of the above

53 Which of the following statements about radiation exposure from CBCT is *true*?
   a Exposure is the same with cephalometric X-rays
   b Exposure is approximately the same as that of full mouth series

c Exposure is equal to that of a medical-grade CT scan

d None of the above statements is true

54 A drug has a FDA PR category C rating. This means that:

a animal studies demonstrate no fetal risk but human studies are inadequate to determine risk

b human studies demonstrate no fetal risk but animal studies are inadequate to determine risk

c human studies demonstrate fetal toxicity but animal studies are inadequate. The benefit of use does not exceed the risk

d animal studies demonstrate fetal toxicity but human studies are inadequate. The benefit of use may exceed the risk

55 Which of the following local anesthetics is a less favorable choice for use during pregnancy?

a Prilocaine

b Mepivacaine

c Lidocaine

d None of the above

56 Which is considered the ideal local anesthetic that can be used safely in pregnancy?

a 2% Lidocaine with 1:100 000 epinephrine

b 0.5% Bupivacaine with 1:200 000 epinephrine

c 3% Mepivacaine

d 4% Prilocaine +/- vasoconstrictor

57 The antibiotic with the most robust safety record in pregnancy is:

a cephalexin

b amoxicillin

c clindamycin

d vancomycin

58 The estolate form of erythromycin is contraindicated in pregnancy because:

a toxic fetal levels can be reached with even the recommended dose

b it is associated with infant low birth weight

c it causes enamel hypoplasia

d it is associated with maternal reversible hepatotoxicity

59 Which of the following analgesics is not considered safe for use in early pregnancy?

a Oral acetaminophen

b Intravenous acetaminophen

c Ibuprofen

d None of the above

60 Which is considered to be a safe combination of acetaminophen with an opioid analgesic?

a Acetaminophen with codeine

b Acetaminophen with hydrocodone

c Acetaminophen with oxycodone

d All of the above

61 The known consequences of smoking during pregnancy include the following conditions *except* for:

a low birth weight

b sudden infant death syndrome

c fluctuating dental asymmetry

d neonatal abstinence syndrome

62 Fetal alcohol syndrome is associated with the following oral conditions *except* for:

a cleft lip and palate

b delayed shedding of primary teeth

c tongue thrust

d prolonged and excessive drooling

63 One of the most common oral conditions resulting from the use of illicit drugs in pregnant and nonpregnant women is xerostomia.

a True

b False

64 Which of the oral sedatives listed below is absolutely contraindicated in pregnancy?

a Diazepam

b Triazolam

c Chlordiazepoxide

d All of the above

65 The N_2O concentrations in dental procedure rooms should be kept at the recommended exposure limit (approximately 55 ppm or 75 milligrams per cubic meter).
a True
b False

66 Which of the following statements about maternal hypercapnia and hypocapnia during procedural IV sedation is *not* true?
a It is tolerated by the fetus
b It causes fetal respiratory acidosis
c It results in uterine artery vasoconstriction
d It depresses the myocardium

67 What is the FDA PR rating of the following procedural IV sedation drugs?
• Fentanyl _____
• Propofol _____
• Ketamine _____
• Midazolam _____

68 Neonatal abstinence syndrome does not only affect infants exposed to illicit sub-

stances, but also infants exposed to the treatments for opioid addictions.
a True
b False

69 Which of the following statements regarding the use of general anesthesia in the pregnant patient is *not* true?
a Teratogenic agents should be avoided
b Premature labor should be prevented
c Fetal monitoring is very rarely required
d Nonreassuring fetal status should be prevented

70 Which is the only antibiotic so far known whose concentrations are higher in the umbilical cord than maternal plasma?
a Cefmenoxime
b Ceftizoxime
c Ampicillin
d Gentamicin

71 MRI is contraindicated in pregnancy because it can cause teratogenicity, fetal tissue heating, and fetal acoustic damage.
a True
b False

Correct Answers and Comments

1 a
2 d
3 c
4 d (Through vasodilation)
5 Aortic <u>augmentation</u> index
6 b
7 c (Through increased bicarbonate excretion from the kidneys)
8 d
9 a (Platelet activation is accelerated potentially at the placental circulation)
10 d
11 c
12 b
13 a
14 b (Is lower)
15 (The current notion is that the maternal immune system is modulated but not suppressed)

16 d
17 c (Tachycardia)*

*Editor's comment: In some literature references, bradycardia is mentioned among the signs and symptoms of SHS. The authors of those articles make reference to the study of Holmes (1960) who studied 500 women pregnant 36 or more weeks for the development of SHS in the supine position. 45 women developed a rise (50% or more) in diastolic pressure in this position but only 3 responded with bradycardia. 31 women with a drop of systolic blood pressure ranging from 30% to 49.9% developed tachycardia whereas 10 women with a drop in systolic pressure >50% after an initial rise (tachycardia) showed a precipitous fall in pulse rate apparently because of fainting as it is reported in the study. Therefore, tachycardia is the predominant cardiovascular response in SHS and not bradycardia.

Holmes F. (1960) Incidence of the supine hypotensive syndrome in late pregnancy. *Journal of Obstetrics and Gynaecology of the British Empire*, **67**, 254.

18 <u>hypoxia</u>
19 c
20 c (The urinary tone is decreased leading in urine stasis which also predisposes to UTIs in pregnancy)
21 7%
22 b (The oral cavity is also affected)
23 d (Impetigo herpetiformis is not a variant of HSV, and the oral cavity involvement is in the form of geographic tongue)
24 <u>49%</u>
25 <u>smells</u>
26 c
27 b (*Streptococcus mutans* and not *Staph. aureus*)
28 c
29 c (Second and third trimesters)
30 c (The amalgam should be well condensed until overfilled and then the mercury-rich layer carved off)
31 <u>oxygen</u> <u>inhibition</u> <u>layer</u>
32 d (The progressive increase in heart rate which peaks in the third trimester may *help* to maintain end-organ perfusion until later stages of septic shock)
33 d
34 c
35 b (The current notion is that the maternal immune system is modulated but not suppressed)
36 d
37 c (Force could have also been applied to the abdomen and hospital referral is justified because complications limited to the pregnancy itself, such as an abruption, can occur after even relatively minor trauma to the abdomen from falls, domestic abuse, and low-speed motor vehicle accidents)
38 a
39 a

40 c (Association of aspirin use with Reye syndrome and potential for bleeding secondary to impaired platelet function. However, maternal ingestion of anti-platelet doses (e.g., 75–100 mg daily) of aspirin during breastfeeding would not be expected to be problematical in healthy term infants)
41 b
42 b
43 b (New AHA recommendations)
44 c
45 d
46 c
47 b (Blood-soaked towels, blood clots, and tissues should be sent to the hospital with the patient so that spontaneous abortion can be confirmed)
48 a (Can cause vaginal bleeding in early pregnancy)
49 d
50 c (False labor)
51 b
52 d
53 b
54 d
55 b
56 a
57 b
58 d (Can cause cholestatic hepatitis)
59 b
60 c (Oxycodone is safer in pregnancy)
61 d
62 a
63 a (Most if not all illicit drugs cause xerostomia)
64 b (Animal studies have shown evidence of retarded or impaired skeletal formation, and impaired viability and weight gain. There are no controlled data in human pregnancy)
65 b (The recommended exposure is approximately 25 ppm or 45 milligrams per cubic meter)
66 a
67 Fentanyl C, Propofol B, Ketamine N (not classified), Midazolam C
68 a
69 c
70 b
71 b

Index

Page locators in **bold** indicate tables. Page locators in *italics* indicate figures.

Dental Management of the Pregnant Patient, First Edition. Edited by Christos A. Skouteris.
© 2018 John Wiley & Sons, Inc. Published 2018 by John Wiley & Sons, Inc.